T0362398

The Gut in MRI: From the Upper to the Lower Digestive Tract

Editor

ANDREA LAGHI

MAGNETIC RESONANCE IMAGING CLINICS OF NORTH AMERICA

www.mri.theclinics.com

Consulting Editors
SURESH K. MUKHERJI
LYNNE S. STEINBACH

February 2020 • Volume 28 • Number 1

ELSEVIER

1600 John F. Kennedy Boulevard • Suite 1800 • Philadelphia, Pennsylvania, 19103-2899

http://www.mri.theclinics.com

MRI CLINICS OF NORTH AMERICA Volume 28, Number 1
February 2020 ISSN 1064-9689, ISBN 13: 978-0-323-75417-0

Editor: John Vassallo (j.vassallo@elsevier.com)
Developmental Editor: Kristen Helm

Magnetic Resonance Imaging Clinics of North America (ISSN 1064-9689) is published quarterly by Elsevier Inc., 360 Park Avenue South, New York, NY 10010-1710. Months of issue are February, May, August, and November. Business and Editorial Offices: 1600 John F. Kennedy Blvd., Ste. 1800, Philadelphia, PA 19103-2899. Customer Service Office: 3251 Riverport Lane, Maryland Heights, MO 63043. Periodicals postage paid at New York, NY and additional mailing offices. Subscription prices are $404.00 per year (domestic individuals), $773.00 per year (domestic institutions), $100.00 per year (domestic students/residents), $437.00 per year (Canadian individuals), $1007.00 per year (Canadian institutions), $550.00 per year (international individuals), $1007.00 per year (international institutions), $100.00 per year (Canadian students/residents), and $275.00 per year (international students/residents). International air speed delivery is included in all *Clinics* subscription prices. All prices are subject to change without notice. **POSTMASTER:** Send address changes to *Magnetic Resonance Imaging Clinics*, Elsevier Health Sciences Division, Subscription Customer Service, 3251 Riverport Lane, Maryland Heights, MO 63043. Customer Service (orders, claims, online, change of address): Elsevier Health Sciences Division, Subscription **Customer Service, 3251 Riverport Lane, Maryland Heights, MO 63043. Tel:1-800-654-2452 (U.S. and Canada); 314-447-8871 (outside U.S. and Canada). Fax: 314-447-8029. E-mail: journalscustomerservice-usa@elsevier.com (for print support); journalsonlinesupport-usa@elsevier.com (for online support).**

Reprints. For copies of 100 or more of articles in this publication, please contact the Commercial Reprints Department, Elsevier Inc., 360 Park Avenue South, New York, NY 10010-1710. Tel.: 212-633-3874; Fax: 212-633-3820; E-mail: reprints@elsevier.com.

Magnetic Resonance Imaging Clinics of North America is covered in the *RSNA Index of Imaging Literature, MEDLINE/PubMed (Index Medicus),* and *EMBASE/Excerpta Medica.*

Contributors

CONSULTING EDITORS

SURESH K. MUKHERJI, MD, MBA, FACR
Clinical Professor, Marian University, Director
of Head and Neck Radiology, ProScan
Imaging, Regional Medical Director, Envision
Physician Services, Carmel, Indiana, USA

LYNNE S. STEINBACH, MD, FACR
Emeritus Professor of Radiology on Full Recall,
Department of Radiology and Biomedical
Imaging, University of California, San
Francisco, San Francisco, California, USA

EDITOR

ANDREA LAGHI, MD
Professor and Chairman of Radiology,
Department of Surgical and Medical Sciences
and Translational Medicine, School of
Medicine and Psychology, "Sapienza"–
University of Rome, Chairman of Radiology
Unit–Sant'Andrea University Hospital, Rome,
Italy

AUTHORS

DANIEL A. ADAMO, MD
Department of Radiology, Mayo Clinic,
Rochester, Minnesota, USA

LUCA ALBARELLO, MD
Department of Pathology, IRCCS San Raffaele
Scientific Institute, Vita-Salute San Raffaele
University, Milan, Italy

FABIO BARRA, MD
Academic Unit of Obstetrics and Gynaecology,
IRCCS Ospedale Policlinico San Martino,
Department of Neurosciences, Rehabilitation,
Ophthalmology, Genetics, Maternal and Child
Health (DiNOGMI), University of Genoa,
Genova, Italy

REGINA BEETS-TAN, MD, PhD
Radiologist, Department of Radiology, The
Netherlands Cancer Institute, Amsterdam, The
Netherlands

ENNIO BISCALDI, MD
Department of Radiology, Galliera Hospital,
Genova, Italy

**DARREN BOONE, MB BS, BSc, MD, MRCP,
FRCR**
Consultant Gastrointestinal and Oncological
Radiologist, Department of Specialist Imaging,
University College London Hospital, London,
United Kingdom

NUNZIA CAPOZZI, MD
Department of Radiology, Hospital Clínic
Barcelona, Barcelona, Catalonia, Spain;
Department of Radiology, Hospital S. Orsola-
Malpighi, University of Bologna, Bologna, Italy

LUÍS CURVO-SEMEDO, MD, PhD
Assistant Professor, University Clinic of
Radiology, Faculty of Medicine, University of
Coimbra, Radiology Consultant, Clinical
Academic Centre of Coimbra, Coimbra,
Portugal

FRANCESCO DE COBELLI, MD
Department of Radiology, Experimental
Imaging Center, IRCCS San Raffaele Scientific
Institute, Vita-Salute San Raffaele University,
Milan, Italy

REBECCA A.P. DIJKHOFF, MD
Department of Internal Medicine, Zuyderland
Medical Centre, Sittard/Heerlen, The
Netherlands

JONATHAN R. DILLMAN, MD
Associate Professor, Department of Radiology,
Cincinnati Children's Hospital, Cincinnati,
Ohio, USA

SIMONE FERRERO, MD, PhD
Academic Unit of Obstetrics and Gynaecology,
IRCCS Ospedale Policlinico San Martino,
Department of Neurosciences, Rehabilitation,
Ophthalmology, Genetics, Maternal and Child
Health (DiNOGMI), University of Genoa,
Genova, Italy

JEFF L. FIDLER, MD
Department of Radiology, Mayo Clinic,
Rochester, Minnesota, USA

JOEL G. FLETCHER, MD
Professor, Department of Radiology, Mayo
Clinic, Rochester, Minnesota, USA

FRANCESCO GIGANTI, MD
Department of Radiology, University College
London Hospital NHS Foundation Trust,
Division of Surgery and Interventional Science,
Faculty of Medical Sciences, University
College London, London, United Kingdom

MARY-LOUISE C. GREER, MBBS
Associate Professor, Department of Medical
Imaging, University of Toronto, Department of
Diagnostic Imaging, The Hospital for Sick
Children, Toronto, Ontario, Canada

GIANFRANCO GUALDI, MD
Radiology Department, Umberto I Hospital
Sapienza University, Rome, Italy

MARIANNA GUIDA, MD
Radiology Department, Umberto I Hospital
Sapienza University, Rome, Italy

LUÍS S. GUIMARÃES, MD, PhD
Assistant Professor, Department of Medical
Imaging, University of Toronto, Joint
Department of Medical Imaging, Sinai Health
System, UHN and Women's College Hospital,
Toronto, Ontario, Canada

**STEVE HALLIGAN, MB BS, MD, PhD, FRCP,
FRCR, FMedSci**
Head, UCL Department of Imaging, Director,
UCL Centre for Medical Imaging, London,
United Kingdom

FRANCESCA LAGHI, MD
Radiology Department, Umberto I Hospital
Sapienza University, Rome, Italy

MONIQUE MAAS, MD, PhD
Radiologist, Department of Radiology, The
Netherlands Cancer Institute, Amsterdam, The
Netherlands

GABRIELE MASSELLI, MD, PhD
Radiology Department, Umberto I Hospital
Sapienza University, Rome, Italy

CHRISTINE O. MENIAS, MD
Department of Radiology, Mayo Clinic,
Phoenix, Arizona, USA

DIEGO PALUMBO, MD
Department of Radiology, Experimental
Imaging Center, IRCCS San Raffaele Scientific
Institute, Vita-Salute San Raffaele University,
Milan, Italy

ELISABETTA POLETTINI, MD
Radiology Department, Umberto I Hospital
Sapienza University, Rome, Italy

JORDI RIMOLA, MD, PhD
Department of Radiology, Hospital Clínic
Barcelona, CIBER-EHD, University of
Barcelona, Barcelona, Catalonia, Spain

RICCARDO ROSATI, MD
Department of Gastrointestinal Surgery,
IRCCS San Raffaele Scientific Institute, Vita-
Salute San Raffaele University, Milan, Italy

SHANNON P. SHEEDY, MD
Department of Radiology, Mayo Clinic,
Rochester, Minnesota, USA

JAAP STOKER, MD, PhD
Radiologist, Department of Radiology and
Nuclear Medicine, Amsterdam UMC, Location
AMC, University of Amsterdam, Amsterdam,
The Netherlands

STUART A. TAYLOR, MB BS, BSc, MD, MRCP, FRCR
Professor of Medical Imaging, Centre for Medical Imaging, University College London, London, United Kingdom

JEROEN A.W. TIELBEEK, MD, PhD
Radiologist, Department of Radiology and Nuclear Medicine, Amsterdam UMC, Location AMC, University of Amsterdam, Amsterdam, The Netherlands

MICHAEL L. WELLS, MD
Department of Radiology, Mayo Clinic, Rochester, Minnesota, USA

Contents

approach for each patient. Magnetic resonance (MR) imaging provides powerful objective insights into the disease process, and its high sensitivity and specificity for detecting inflammation make it essential for diagnosis and management. Growing evidence indicates that MR provides reliable and accurate information that enables detection of changes after treatment with biological drugs. This article provides an overview of currently established and emerging MR biomarkers for assessing response to treatment in patients with CD.

MR enterography is frequently ordered for patients with suspected small bowel disorders. In this article, disease-causing malabsorption, vasculitides, and some of the less common small bowel diseases are reviewed. The clinical presentations, diagnostic criteria, and imaging findings of these diseases are discussed. Because the imaging findings in several small bowel diseases are nonspecific and/or overlap, radiologists must correlate clinical data with imaging to develop a narrower differential diagnosis. The unique or characteristic findings in certain diseases are also emphasized.

Tumors of the small intestine represent less than 5% of all gastrointestinal tract neoplasms. Magnetic resonance (MR) imaging is rapidly increasing clinical acceptance to evaluate the small bowel and can be the initial imaging method to investigate small bowel diseases. MR examinations may provide the first opportunity to detect and characterize tumors of the small bowel. Intraluminal and extraluminal MR findings, combined with contrast enhancement and functional information, allow accurate diagnoses and consequently characterization of small bowel neoplasms. This article describes the MR findings of primary small bowel neoplasms and the MR findings for the differential diagnosis are discussed.

Intestinal endometriosis occurs in 4% to 37% of women with deep endometriosis (DE). Noninvasive diagnosis of presence and characteristics of rectosigmoid endometriosis permits the best counseling of patients and ensures best therapeutic planning. Magnetic resonance enema (MR-e) is accurate in diagnosing DE. After colon cleansing, rectal distention and opacification improves the performance of MR-e in diagnosing rectosigmoid endometriosis. MR imaging cannot optimally assess the depth of penetration of endometriosis in the intestinal wall. There is a need for multicentric studies with a larger sample size to evaluate reproducibility of MR-e in diagnosis of rectosigmoid endometriosis for less experienced radiologists.

The imaging of rectal cancer has evolved noticeably over the past 2 decades, paralleling the advances in therapy. The methods for imaging rectal cancer are increasingly used in clinical practice with the purpose of helping to detect, characterize and stage rectal cancer. In this setting, MR imaging emerged as the most useful imaging method for primary staging of rectal cancer; the present review focuses on the role of MR imaging in this regard.

Rectal Cancer: Assessing Response to Neoadjuvant Therapy   117

Monique Maas, Rebecca A.P. Dijkhoff, and Regina Beets-Tan

MR imaging plays a crucial role in the post-CRT assessment of rectal cancer; results are used for treatment planning. Radiologists should assess response or progression, possibility of a complete response, risk factors for incomplete resection, and nodal stage. T2-weighted MR imaging with diffusion-weighted imaging yields the best results to identify a complete response, but endoscopy is also very important. Overstaging of transmural and MRF invasion after CRT occur regularly, owing to residual stranding regarded as tumor to err on the safe side. Nodal restaging is a challenge. A structured report format or checklist is recommended.

Staging of Anal Cancer: Role of MR Imaging   127

Monique Maas, Jeroen A.W. Tielbeek, and Jaap Stoker

Anal cancer is a relatively rare malignancy. Treatment consists of chemoradiation and most patients achieve a complete response. Local evaluation of the T and N stage is performed by MR imaging. Whole-body staging with 18F-fluorodesoxyglucose positron emission tomography computed tomography scans or computed tomography scans is used to detect metastases. T stage is based on tumor size or invasion of organs. N stage is based on nodal location. After chemoradiation, clinical evaluation and MR imaging is used to assess tumor and nodal response. Maximal response is achieved 6 months after chemoradiation. Beware of development of anal cancer in perianal fistulas.

Magnetic Resonance Imaging of Fistula-In-Ano   141

Steve Halligan

This article explains the pathogenesis of fistula-in-ano and details the different classifications of fistula encountered, describe their features on MR imaging, and explains how imaging influences subsequent surgical treatment and ultimate clinical outcome. Precise preoperative characterization of the anatomic course of the fistula and all associated infection via MR imaging is critical for surgery to be most effective. MR imaging is the preeminent imaging modality used to answer pertinent surgical questions.

MAGNETIC RESONANCE IMAGING CLINICS OF NORTH AMERICA

SERIES OF RELATED INTEREST

Neuroimaging Clinics of North America
Available at: www.neuroimaging.theclinics.com

PET Clinics
Available at: www.pet.theclinics.com

Radiologic Clinics of North America
Available at: www.radiologic.theclinics.com

VISIT THE CLINICS ONLINE!
Access your subscription at:
www.theclinics.com

PROGRAM OBJECTIVE

The goal of *Magnetic Resonance Imaging Clinics of North America* is to keep practicing physicians up to date with current clinical practice by providing timely articles reviewing the state of the art in patient care.

TARGET AUDIENCE

All practicing physicians and healthcare professionals who provide patient care utilizing findings from Magnetic Resonance Imaging.

LEARNING OBJECTIVES

Upon completion of this activity, participants will be able to:
1. Review the role of MRI for the diagnosis of rectal cancer and patient management.
2. Discuss the role of MRI in the evaluation of prognosis and treatment response in patients with esophageal and gastric cancers.
3. Recognize the role of MR in the diagnosis and classification of Crohn's Disease, as well as assessing response to therapy.

ACCREDITATION

The Elsevier Office of Continuing Medical Education (EOCME) is accredited by the Accreditation Council for Continuing Medical Education (ACCME) to provide continuing medical education for physicians.

The EOCME designates this journal-based CME activity enduring material for a maximum of 11 *AMA PRA Category 1 Credit*(s)™. Physicians should claim only the credit commensurate with the extent of their participation in the activity.

All other healthcare professionals requesting continuing education credit for this enduring material will be issued a certificate of participation.

DISCLOSURE OF CONFLICTS OF INTEREST

The EOCME assesses conflict of interest with its instructors, faculty, planners, and other individuals who are in a position to control the content of CME activities. All relevant conflicts of interest that are identified are thoroughly vetted by EOCME for fair balance, scientific objectivity, and patient care recommendations. EOCME is committed to providing its learners with CME activities that promote improvements or quality in healthcare and not a specific proprietary business or a commercial interest.

The planning committee, staff, authors and editors listed below have identified no financial relationships or relationships to products or devices they or their spouse/life partner have with commercial interest related to the content of this CME activity:

Daniel A. Adamo, MD; Luca Albarello, MD; Fabio Barra, MD; Regina Beets-Tan, MD, PhD; Ennio Biscaldi, MD; Darren Boone, MB BS, BSc, MD, MRCP, FRCR; Nunzia Capozzi, MD; Luís Curvo-Semedo, MD, PhD; Francesco De Cobelli, MD; Rebecca A.P. Dijkhoff, MD; Jonathan R. Dillman, MD; Simone Ferrero, MD, PhD; Jeff L. Fidler, MD; Joel G. Fletcher, MD; Francesco Giganti, MD; Mary-Louise C. Greer, MBBS; Gianfranco Gualdi, MD; Marianna Guida, MD; Luís S. Guimarães, MD, PhD; Steve Halligan, MB BS, MD, PhD, FRCP, FRCR, FMedSci; Alison Kemp; Pradeep Kuttysankaran; Francesca Laghi, MD; Andrea Laghi, MD, PhD; Monique Maas, MD, PhD; Gabriele Masselli, MD, PhD; Christine O. Menias, MD; Suresh K. Mukherji, MD, MBA, FACR; Diego Palumbo, MD; Elisabetta Polettini, MD; Jordi Rimola, MD, PhD; Riccardo Rosati, MD; Shannon P. Sheedy, MD; Lynne S. Steinbach, MD, FACR; Jaap Stoker, MD, PhD; Jeroen A.W. Tielbeek, MD, PhD; John Vassallo; Michael L. Wells, MD.

The planning committee, staff, authors and editors listed below have identified financial relationships or relationships to products or devices they or their spouse/life partner have with commercial interest related to the content of this CME activity:

Stuart A. Taylor, MB BS, BSc, MD, MRCS, FRCR: consultant/advisor for Robarts Clinical Trials and owns stock in Motilinet.

UNAPPROVED/OFF-LABEL USE DISCLOSURE

The EOCME requires CME faculty to disclose to the participants:
1. When products or procedures being discussed are off-label, unlabelled, experimental, and/or investigational (not US Food and Drug Administration [FDA] approved); and
2. Any limitations on the information presented, such as data that are preliminary or that represent ongoing research, interim analyses, and/or unsupported opinions. Faculty may discuss information about pharmaceutical agents that is outside of FDA-approved labelling. This information is intended solely for CME and is not intended to promote off-label use of these medications. If you have any questions, contact the medical affairs department of the manufacturer for the most recent prescribing information.

TO ENROLL

To enroll in the *Magnetic Resonance Imaging Clinics of North America* Continuing Medical Education program, call customer service at 1-800-654-2452 or sign up online at http://www.theclinics.com/home/cme. The CME program is available to subscribers for an additional annual fee of USD 260.

METHOD OF PARTICIPATION

In order to claim credit, participants must complete the following:

1. Complete enrolment as indicated above.
2. Read the activity.
3. Complete the CME Test and Evaluation. Participants must achieve a score of 70% on the test. All CME Tests and Evaluations must be completed online.

CME INQUIRIES/SPECIAL NEEDS

For all CME inquiries or special needs, please contact elsevierCME@elsevier.com.

Foreword

The Gut in MR Imaging: From the Upper to the Lower Digestive Tract

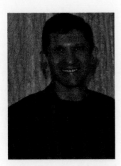

Suresh K. Mukherji, MD, MBA, FACR
Consulting Editor

I can honestly say that I knew nothing about MR imaging of the gut...until now! Thank you Dr Andrea Laghi for creating such a wonderful issue covering such a challenging topic. There are specific topics devoted to disorders of esophagus, stomach, small bowel, large bowel, and the anorectal region. The articles focused on cancer staging will be especially helpful for all individuals involved in care of these very complex malignancies. I want to thank all of the authors for their wonderful contributions. Your efforts are deeply appreciated.

On a personnel note, I met Andrea on a Radiological Society of North America Visiting Professor trip to Kampala, Uganda in early 2018. In fact, he and I were roommates for 2 weeks! We shared an incredible educational and cultural experience, which included a land and water safari. Our hosts were fantastic, and attendees were incredibly welcoming. He and I became

fast friends, and I was very happy when he accepted this invitation to edit an issue covering MR of the large and small bowel. This issue is innovative, interesting, and relevant, which are the 3 objectives he hoped to accomplish. Andrea, thank you very much for your wonderful contribution and friendship!

Suresh K. Mukherji, MD, MBA, FACR
Clinical Professor
Marian University
Director of Head & Neck Radiology
ProScan Imaging
Regional Medical Director
Envision Physician Services
Carmel, Indiana, USA

E-mail address:
sureshmukherji@hotmail.com

Magn Reson Imaging Clin N Am 28 (2020) xiii
https://doi.org/10.1016/j.mric.2019.09.008
1064-9689/20/© 2019 Published by Elsevier Inc.

Foreword

The Gut in MR Imaging: From the Upper to the Lower Digestive Tract

Preface
The Gut in MR Imaging: A Successful Story

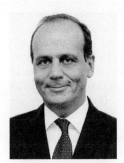

Andrea Laghi, MD
Editor

The decision regarding the topic of a new issue of *Magnetic Resonance Imaging Clinics of North America* is not simple, both for the publisher and for the editor. The topic must be innovative, attractive to the reader, and useful in routine practice. Does the topic "the gut in MR imaging" fulfill these important criteria? I am personally convinced of this, and I hope the readers of this issue will also be.

Through the various articles, we tried to touch the most relevant aspects concerning the use of MR imaging for gut imaging, from the study technique to the clinical applications, common and not.

Following an anatomic path, the first organs were the esophagus and the stomach. Esophago-gastric MR imaging is still a niche application, because imaging protocols are not standardized yet, but extremely promising, especially in oncology. The images presented by the authors demonstrate the diagnostic value of MR imaging, if properly performed. Moreover, since neoadjuvant therapy is becoming routine in many patients affected by esophageal and gastric cancers, MR imaging can offer quantitative imaging biomarkers (still under investigation) for the evaluation of prognosis and treatment response.

A larger space was devoted to the small intestine, which finds in MR imaging an indispensable study technique. This is the reason an entire article is dedicated to the current consensus statements from the United States and Europe, which have recently been published to inform evidence-based small bowel MR imaging technique. MR imaging of the small bowel is crucial, in particular, in Crohn disease. Diagnosis and disease balance of Crohn, in fact, are based not only on histology but also on cross-sectional imaging, in particular, MR imaging. MR imaging is more panoramic than ultrasound and is noninvasive compared with computed tomography (CT). MR imaging is much more than US and CT because it is multiparametric and, thus, it offers a better evaluation of inflammation and, in the near future, fibrosis. MR imaging is functional and can investigate bowel motility. And last, but not least, quantitative scores make MR a potential imaging biomarker in the assessment of therapy response, which is extremely important in the era of biologic drugs.

To cover the entire spectrum of small bowel diseases, the next 2 articles are dedicated to malabsorption syndromes, vasculitis, ischemia, malignancy-associated conditions, and tumors. The more frequently small bowel MR imaging investigations are performed, the higher the possibility of encountering these uncommon entities.

When approaching the large bowel, we have focused our attention on the clinically relevant applications of MR imaging. We omitted magnetic resonance (MR) colonography on purpose. MR colonography, despite being around for more than a decade, has not found a position yet, probably because of the success of CT colonography. The assessment of large bowel involvement in deep pelvic endometriosis is becoming a common examination, because of the awareness of the disease of female patients and the need of reducing invasive diagnostic procedures like laparoscopy.

Magn Reson Imaging Clin N Am 28 (2020) xv–xvi
https://doi.org/10.1016/j.mric.2019.09.007
1064-9689/20/© 2019 Published by Elsevier Inc.

In rectal cancer, the role of MR imaging is crucial, not only for diagnosis, but particularly for patient management: it is on the basis of MR imaging that the rectal tumor board will decide the most appropriate therapy and will inform the patient about his prognosis. MR imaging performed following neoadjuvant therapy will contribute to the decision if resecting the patient or referring him to a "watch-and-wait" strategy. Anal cancer follows a similar diagnostic strategy: MR imaging at the time of the diagnosis and for the assessment of the response to chemoradiotherapy. The last article is dedicated to anal fistulas, a common entity where MR, in complex cases, is the best modality to describe the anatomic course of the fistula, and it is critical for the success of surgery.

I would like to thank the authors of the articles for their excellent and invaluable contributions. It was certainly a great effort, and the readers will be rewarded by the result.

Andrea Laghi, MD
Department of Surgical and Medical Sciences
and Translational Medicine
School of Medicine and Psychology
"Sapienza"–University of Rome
Sant'Andrea University Hospital
Via di Grottarossa, 1035-1039
00189 Rome, Italy

E-mail address:
andrea.laghi@uniroma1.it

Esophagus and Stomach
Is There a Role for MR Imaging?

Francesco De Cobelli, MD[a,b,*], Diego Palumbo, MD[a,b,1], Luca Albarello, MD[b,c,1], Riccardo Rosati, MD[b,d,1], Francesco Giganti, MD[e,f]

KEYWORDS

- Esophageal cancer • Gastric cancer • Magnetic resonance imaging • Staging
- Treatment response • Prognosis

KEY POINTS

- MR imaging can be included in the diagnostic pathway of a wide range of benign and malignant conditions of the esophagus and the stomach.
- An adequate MR imaging protocol is crucial for the assessment of the esophagus and stomach. This includes high-resolution multiplanar T2-weighted, diffusion-weighted, and dynamic contrast-enhanced imaging.
- There remains a need for improvement and standardization before MR imaging becomes an accepted and widely adopted method to investigate the gastroesophageal tract.
- Different quantitative imaging biomarkers from DWI and DCE hold promise in the evaluation of the aggressiveness, treatment response and prognosis of esophageal and gastric cancer.

INTRODUCTION

A wide range of esophageal and gastric conditions (both benign and malignant) can be investigated with endoscopy or barium contrast studies for the evaluation of mucosal surface lesions; such techniques, however, provide little or no information about the extramucosal extent of disease.

Other imaging modalities, that is, endoscopic ultrasound (EUS), computed tomography (CT), and ^{18}F-fluorodeoxyglucose (^{18}F-FDG) PET permit the assessment of parietal and extraparietal involvement, lymphadenopathies, and distant metastases.

Over the last 20 years, MR imaging has been increasingly used as a valid diagnostic tool in adjunct to these imaging techniques.

In this article, the authors provide the reader with some of the most common MR imaging findings in the gastroesophageal tract and discuss the goals for a widespread application of this technique at this regard.

MR IMAGING TECHNIQUE

MR imaging is performed with either a 1.5 T or 3 T system, using an external surface coil (ie, multiple-channel phased array cardiac coil) with cardiac and respiratory triggering.

MR imaging of the esophagus does not require any specific preparation apart from the administration of intramuscular scopolamine (in the absence of contraindications), especially when

Disclosure: F. Giganti is funded by the UCL Graduate Research Scholarship and the Brahm PhD scholarship in memory of Chris Adams. The other authors have nothing to disclose.

[a] Department of Radiology, Experimental Imaging Center, IRCCS San Raffaele Scientific Institute, Milan, Italy; [b] Vita-Salute San Raffaele University, Milan, Italy; [c] Department of Pathology, IRCCS San Raffaele Scientific Institute, Milan, Italy; [d] Department of Gastrointestinal Surgery, IRCCS San Raffaele Scientific Institute, Milan, Italy; [e] Department of Radiology, University College London Hospital NHS Foundation Trust, London, UK; [f] Division of Surgery and Interventional Science, Faculty of Medical Sciences, University College London, 3rd Floor, Charles Bell House, 43-45 Foley Street, London W1W 7TS, UK

[1] Present address: Via Olgettina 60, Milan 20132, Italy.

* Corresponding author. Via Olgettina 60, Milan 20132, Italy.

E-mail address: decobelli.francesco@hsr.it

Magn Reson Imaging Clin N Am 28 (2020) 1–15
https://doi.org/10.1016/j.mric.2019.08.001

the gastroesophageal junction is the anatomic region of interest.

Differently from the esophagus, MR imaging of the stomach requires accurate patient preparation: in particular, proper visceral distension is fundamental to depict the multilayer pattern of the gastric wall.

After a 6-hour fasting, distension is obtained by oral administration of at least 500 mL of water immediately before the examination and an intramuscular injection of scopolamine is usually administered to decrease bowel peristalsis.[1–4] Some authors suggest the use of effervescent granules to obtain gastric distension but in our experience it is not generally used, owing to the risk of increasing air artifacts from the gastric lumen.[1–4]

When water is used as oral contrast agent, the patient is scanned in the prone or supine position dependent on the location of the region of interest to allow proper contact between the oral contrast medium and the visceral wall. The positions should be reversed when effervescent granules are used.[1]

Although standardized MR imaging protocols for both organs have yet to be reported, as a rule of thumb the examination should include:

- High-resolution multiplanar T2-weighted imaging (T2-WI), including turbo spin echo sequences with and without fat suppression with cardiac and respiratory gating.

T2-WI is crucial for the anatomy of the organ, as it allows excellent soft-tissue contrast together with good spatial resolution and a high signal-to-noise ratio:

- Axial diffusion-weighted imaging (DWI) with different b values (usually up to 1000 s/mm^2).

DWI provides information about the tissue structure and cellular density because it reflects the mobility of water protons measuring the apparent diffusion coefficient (ADC). This quantitative index is considered a promising imaging biomarker both for the esophagus and the stomach[5,6]:

- Axial breath-hold T1-weighted sequences with fat suppression, acquired before and after intravenous injection of contrast agent.

Dynamic contrast enhanced (DCE) MR imaging involves the acquisition of serial T1-weighted images before and after injection of a bolus of chelated gadolinium molecule. The application of DCE-MR imaging in oncology has been increasing over the last few years thanks to continuous technical developments. Moreover, different quantitative biomarkers extrapolated from DCE-MR imaging maps according to the

Tofts model have been investigated in the gastroesophageal tract.[7]

Tables 1 and **2** list the 2 protocols for MR imaging of the esophagus and the stomach, respectively. As far as the esophagus is concerned, the study should commence with a sagittal high-resolution T2-weighted acquisition to orientate the axial images perpendicular to the long axis of the organ. A coronal acquisition should be also added in the protocol if the region of interest is the gastroesophageal junction, because this allows to clearly delineate the diaphragmatic hiatus.[6,8]

MR IMAGING ANATOMY
Esophagus

The esophagus is a muscular tube (20–25 cm in length) that connects the pharynx to the stomach and is composed of 3 segments: cervical, thoracic, and abdominal.

Histologically, it is composed of different layers:

- The inner layer (ie, stratified squamous epithelium that changes abruptly at the cardia of the stomach into simple columnar epithelium)
- The muscularis mucosae
- The submucosa
- The inner circular muscular layer
- The outer longitudinal muscular layer

There is no serosal layer and the thickness of the esophageal wall is usually considered physiologic up to 5 mm.

On T1-weighted imaging, the esophagus appears as a structure of low-signal intensity, contrasted by the high-signal intensity of the surrounding fat. The esophageal layers are clearly visible on high-resolution T2-WI MR imaging. On an axial T2-WI acquisition, this is characterized by a 3-layered pattern, the distinction of which is mainly based on the higher signal intensity of the middle layer (**Fig. 1**)[8,9]:

- Mucosa (inner layer): intermediate/low signal-intensity
- Submucosa: high-signal intensity
- Muscularis propria (outer layer): low-signal intensity

There is also evidence of ex vivo studies conducted at 7T demonstrating up to 8 layers of the esophageal wall on ultra-high-resolution T2-weighted sequences.[10]

Stomach

The gastric wall consists of the following 5 layers:

- Mucosa (inner layer)
- Submucosa

Table 1
MR imaging protocol for the esophagus

Parameters	SS Fat-Suppressed T$_2$-Weighted	T$_2$-Weighted	SS EP Diffusion-Weighted[a]	Gadolinium Contrast-Enhanced	TSE PD-BB
Plane	Axial and sagittal/coronal	Axial	Axial	Axial	Sagittal
TR (ms)	Shortest	2400	Single heartbeat	Shortest	1600 (2 heartbeat)
TE (ms)	100	80	58	Shortest	10
Slice thickness (mm)	4	4	4	25	6
Slice gap (mm)	1	0.4	1	Over contiguous slice	–
Matrix size (reconstructed)	320	288	336	288	512
Field of view (mm)	365 × 284	300 × 280	365 × 319	365 × 289	350 × 350
Flip angle (°)	90	90	90	10	90
Acquisition time (s)	14	150[b]	104[b]	94	11
Number of slices	35	18	30	65	10

Abbreviations: EP, echo planar; SS, single shot; TE, echo time; TR, repetition time.
[a] $b = 0, 600$ s/mm^2.
[b] Total duration according to the cardiac and respiratory frequency.

- Muscularis propria
- Subserosa
- Serosa (outer layer)

However, on T2-WI acquired at 1.5 T, the gastric wall is generally depicted as a 3-layer structure, because the muscularis propria, the subserosa, and the serosa are not clearly distinguishable[11]:

- Mucosa: low-signal intensity
- Submucosa: intermediate- to high-signal intensity

Table 2
MR imaging protocol for the stomach

Parameters	SS Fat-Suppressed T$_2$-Weighted	T$_2$-Weighted	SS EP Diffusion-Weighted[a]	Gadolinium Contrast-Enhanced
Plane	Axial and coronal	Axial	Axial	Axial
TR (ms)	Shortest	2400	Single heartbeat	Shortest
TE (ms)	100	80	58	Shortest
Slice thickness (mm)	4	5	4	25
Slice gap (mm)	1	0.8	1	Over contiguous slice
Matrix size (reconstructed)	336	288	336	288
Field of view (mm)	365 × 284	300 × 280	365 × 319	365 × 289
Flip angle (°)	90	90	90	10
Acquisition time (s)	14	150[b]	104[b]	94
Number of slices	35	18	30	65

Abbreviations: EP, echo planar; SS, single shot; TE, echo time; TR, repetition time.
[a] $b = 0, 600$ s/mm^2.
[b] Total duration according to the cardiac and respiratory frequency.

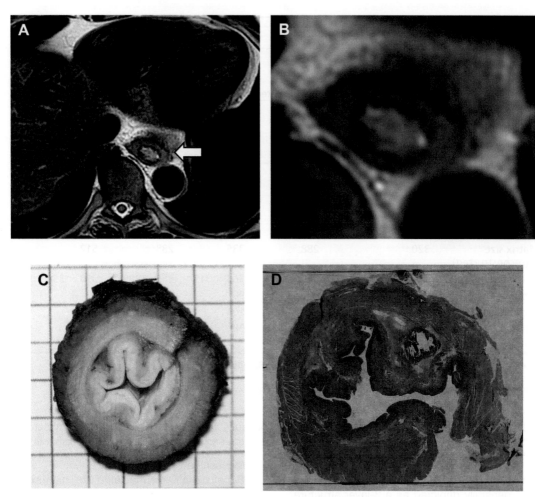

Fig. 1. MR imaging and histology of the normal esophageal wall (*arrow*). Axial T2-weighted (*A*, *B*) images, (*C*) macroscopic, and (*D*) microscopic sections of the resected specimen.

- Outer layer (corresponding to the muscularis propria, the subserosa, and the serosa): low-signal intensity

After intravenous administration of a contrast agent, the normal gastric wall demonstrates a 2-layer pattern, corresponding to the inner mucosal layer (early enhancement) and the outer submucosal and muscular layers (delayed enhancement)[12] (**Fig. 2**).

Regarding the stomach, there are experimental studies on ex vivo specimens with variable magnetic fields demonstrating up to 7 gastric wall layers on T2-WI.[13–15]

MR IMAGING OF THE MOST COMMON BENIGN FINDINGS

In this section, we review the clinical characteristics and MR appearances of the most common

esophageal and gastric benign findings, with emphasis on the MR imaging features.

Esophagus

Esophageal diverticulum

Esophageal diverticula may be formed either by pulsion (ie, increased intraluminal pressure against a weak esophageal wall, more common in the cervical or distal segments) or by traction (eg, scarring, fibrosis, or inflammation in periesophageal tissue, more common in the middle segment). Pulsion diverticula consist only of mucosa (false diverticula), whereas traction diverticula contain all esophageal layers (true diverticula), including muscular layers, and therefore they tend to empty when the esophagus collapses.

According to their location, the most common pulsion diverticula occur at the pharyngoesophageal junction (eg, Zenker's diverticulum) (**Fig. 3**)

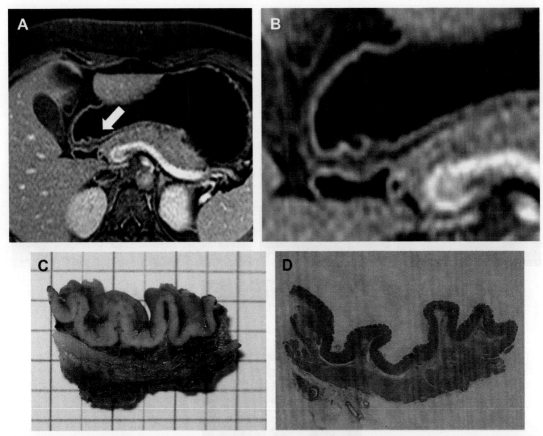

Fig. 2. MR imaging and histology of the normal gastric wall (*arrow*). Axial T1-weighted (*A, B*) images after injection of gadolinium, (*C*) macroscopic, and (*D*) microscopic sections of the resected specimen.

and above the esophageal hiatus (eg, epiphrenic diverticulum).

Esophageal leiomyoma

Leiomyomas are the most common mesenchymal tumors of the esophagus and they can be associated with Alport syndrome.[16] They arise from the smooth muscle layers (usually the muscularis propria) and are mostly found in the middle and distal third of the esophagus (where the content of smooth muscle is greater). They usually range from 2 to 6 cm in diameter and symptoms include dysphagia, vomiting, and weight loss.[17]

On MR imaging, leiomyomas appear as round/ovoid masses with smooth margins, and the surrounding fat is usually preserved. On T1-WI, leiomyomas are usually hyperintense, whereas on T2-WI, they are hypointense to isointense (with respect to the normal esophageal wall) and present homogenous enhancement after administration of contrast medium (**Fig. 4**).[16,18]

However, CT has a higher sensitivity than MR imaging for the detection of esophageal

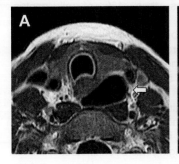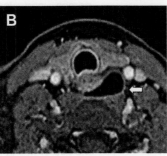

Fig. 3. Zenker's diverticulum in a 44-year-old woman. (*A*) Axial T2-weighted and (*B*) dynamic contrast enhanced images showing left posterolateral outpouching (*arrows*) of the esophageal mucosa and submucosa proximal to the upper esophageal sphincter.

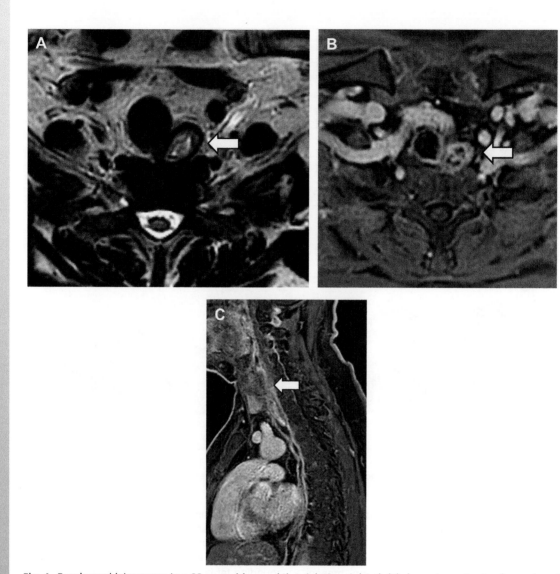

Fig. 4. Esophageal leiomyoma in a 33-year-old man. (*A*) Axial T2-weighted, (*B*) dynamic contrast enhanced, and (*C*) postgadolinium sagittal T1-weighted images showing a submucosal broad-based mass (*arrows*) arising from the left posterior aspect of the esophageal wall and bulging into the esophageal lumen.

leiomyomas, because it is possible to depict the characteristic intratumoral "pop-corn like" calcifications. Surgical resection is the only curative treatment.[19]

Duplication cyst

Esophageal duplication cysts occur almost always in the lower third and on the right aspect of the esophagus, and a clear communication with the esophageal lumen is demonstrated in approximately 20% of cases.[20] On MR imaging, duplication cysts usually show the common features of cysts (ie, hyperintense signal on T2-WI and variable signal intensity on T1-WI, depending on the content) (**Fig. 5**).

Stomach

Gastric lipoma

Gastric lipomas are rare tumors, accounting for only about 5% of the gastrointestinal tract lipomas and less than 1% of all gastric neoplasms.[21,22]

Lipomas are submucosal, well-defined masses (net margins and broad base) composed of mature adipocytes surrounded by a fibrous capsule. They tend to occur as solitary lesions, usually in the gastric antrum.

CT is the imaging examination of choice for gastric lipomas and even though MR imaging is as specific as CT in diagnosing gastric lipomas, the use of MR imaging has been limited.[21,22]

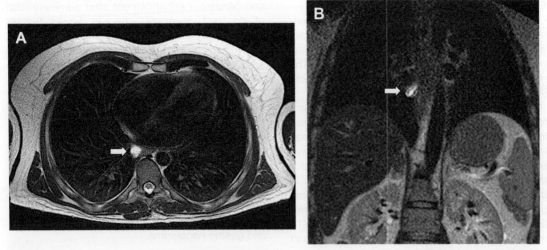

Fig. 5. Incidental finding of an esophageal duplication cyst in a 41-year-old man. (*A*) Axial and (*B*) coronal T2-weighted images show a small mass with cystic MR features (*arrow*) on the right lateral of the distal esophagus.

MR imaging is extremely sensitive to fat and can be of help in confirming the adipose nature of the lesion. Therefore, lipomas show high-signal intensity on T1-WI and low-signal intensity on both T1-WI and T2-WI with fat suppression, with a clear delineation of the gastric wall.

No enhancement is observed after administration of contrast (**Fig. 6**).

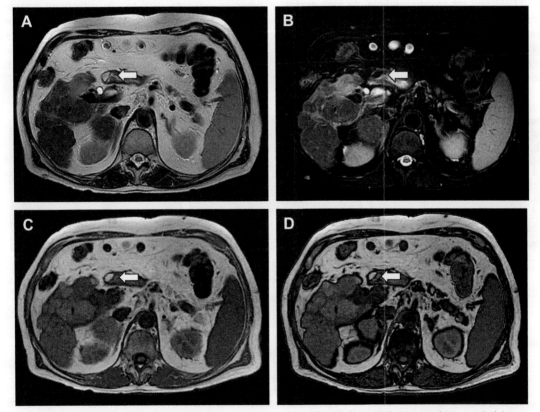

Fig. 6. Incidental finding of a gastric lipoma in a 73-year-old man with liver cirrhosis. Axial T2-weighted images (*A*) without and (*B*) with fat suppression and T1-weighted (*C*) in-phase and (*D*) out-of-phase acquisitions showing a small submucosal mass (*arrows*) in the gastric antrum that contains adipose tissue.

Gastrointestinal stromal tumor

Gastrointestinal stromal tumors (GISTs) are mesen-chymal tumors that arise in the gastrointestinal tract as well as in extravisceral locations, such as the mesentery, omentum, or retroperitoneum. The most common location (70%) is the stomach; 90% of gastric GISTs are benign.[23,24]

Tumor location within the stomach is important for the differential diagnosis: GISTs are often located in the body (75% of cases), whereas leiomyomas and lipomas are almost always seen in the cardia and in the antrum, respec-tively. GISTs differ from leiomyomas in that they derive from a precursor of intestinal pacemaker cells (ie, cells of Cajal) rather than from smooth muscle cells. GISTs may appear as endogastric or exogastric, and they become symptomatic if they enlarge, causing vomiting and ulceration of the lesion (hematemesis, melena, and iron-deficiency anemia).[24]

Small and asymptomatic lesions can be followed-up, but if they are greater than 2 cm they should be surgically removed because there is an increased risk of malignancy.

On MR imaging, GISTs are typically hypointense on T1-WI and return intermediate- to high-signal intensity on T2-WI with respect to the normal gastric wall, and this feature should be considered pathognomonic of GIST (**Fig. 7**).

As far as the enhancement pattern is con-cerned, small GISTs (<5 cm) show homogeneous and persistent enhancement after administration of contrast medium, whereas larger tumors (>5 cm) demonstrate heterogeneous enhance-ment associated with cystic changes, necrosis, and ulceration. Multiplanar acquisitions are crucial to assess the anatomic relationships of GISTs with other organs. There is evidence that DWI is related to degree of malignancy for GISTs, as ADC values are negatively corre-lated with the biological aggressiveness of GISTs.

MR IMAGING FOR MALIGNANT CONDITIONS

Imaging may be helpful for detection, diagnosis, staging, and treatment planning of esophageal and gastric neoplasms.

Esophagus

Esophageal cancer

Esophageal cancer is the ninth most common type of cancer and the sixth most leading cause of cancer-related death.[25]

The 2 major histologic subtypes are squamous cell carcinoma and adenocarcinoma. Early-stage disease can be treated with immediate surgery, whereas patients with locally advanced cancer usually benefit from radiotherapy and chemo-therapy. Therefore, accurate staging is crucial to choose the optimal treatment strategy and to pre-dict the response to neoadjuvant treatment. Several imaging techniques, including EUS, CT,

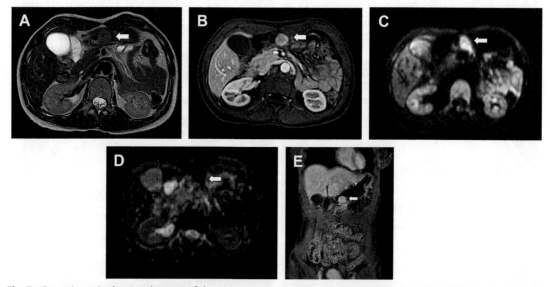

Fig. 7. Gastrointestinal stromal tumor of the greater curvature in a 39-year-old woman. (*A*) Axial T2-weighted, (*B*) dynamic contrast enhanced, (*C*) diffusion-weighted, (*D*) ADC map, and (*E*) coronal postgadolinium T1-weighted images showing a lesion (*arrows*) with equal to high-signal intensity (with respect to the normal gastric wall) on T2-weighted imaging and strong, persistent enhancement after gadolinium.

and ^{18}F-FDG PET, have been investigated in the diagnostic pathway of esophageal cancer.[26] MR imaging is considered a promising technique thanks to the multiplanar acquisitions and the ability to provide excellent soft-tissue contrast, although motion artifacts and the long acquisition time still represent significant technical challenges.[26,27]

On MR imaging, esophageal carcinoma returns intermediate signal intensity on T2-WI, but it should be kept in mind that fibrosis after neoadjuvant therapy may produce a similar appearance. Although MR imaging is not the first choice for staging, it is comparable with CT in determining the resectability, mediastinal invasion, nodal involvement, and presence of distant metastases[28] (**Fig. 8**).

There is also growing evidence of the promising role of MR imaging (especially DWI) in the evaluation of treatment response and prognosis of esophageal cancer[27,29,30] (**Fig. 9**).

Tumor recurrence after surgery
Despite the widespread use of neoadjuvant therapy for locally advanced disease, tumor recurrence after esophagectomy is still common, with a recurrence rate after curative esophagectomy with lymphadenectomy ranging from 40% to 50%.[31]

Recurrence is generally detected as an intraluminal mass or focal wall thickening at the site of the anastomosis.[32] It has been shown that MR imaging is superior to CT for the assessment of local recurrence, given its capability to differentiate between neoplastic tissue and fibrotic scar according to the different MR signal intensities and morphologic criteria (ie, mass effect and loss of fat planes).[32]

On MR imaging, recurrent disease returns increased signal on T2-WI and avid enhancement after administration of contrast, whereas fibrosis is characterized by low signal on T2-WI and weak enhancement (**Fig. 10**).

Stomach

Gastric cancer
Gastric cancer is one of the most common malignancies worldwide.[33]

Accurate preoperative staging of local invasion and nodal involvement is crucial to determine the most appropriate treatment and prognosis for patients with gastric cancer.

Over the last 20 years, multiple imaging techniques (EUS, CT, and PET) have gained importance in the management of gastric cancer by improving the likelihood of a radical tumor resection and overall survival.

Traditionally, the role of MR imaging for gastric cancer has been limited, owing to the relatively long acquisition times, high costs, and technical challenges because of the presence of peristalsis and respiratory artifacts.[3]

However, many technical improvements (ie, fast imaging and motion compensation techniques combined with the use of

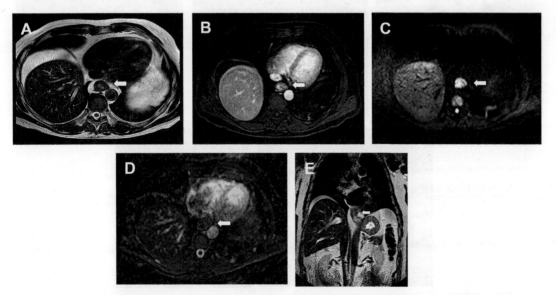

Fig. 8. Lesion involving the distal part of the esophagus in a 66-year-old man. The arrows indicate a slight thickening of the esophageal wall on (A) axial T2-weighted, (B) dynamic contrast enhanced, (C) diffusion-weighted imaging, (D) ADC map, and (E) coronal T2-weighted images. The ADC value of the lesion was 1.58×10^{-3} mm^2/s. Final pathology demonstrated esophageal adenocarcinoma (pT3N1).

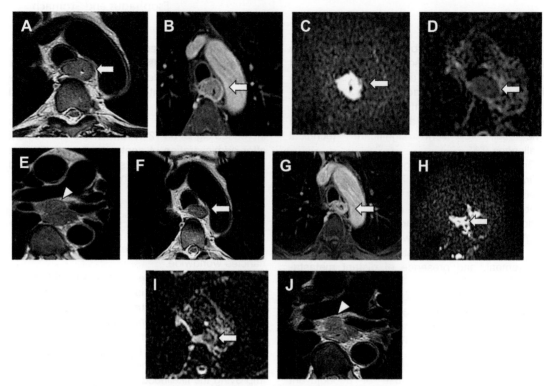

Fig. 9. Lesion of the middle part of the esophagus in a 59-year-old man (*A–E*) before and (*F–J*) after neoadjuvant chemoradiotherapy. The arrows indicate thickening of the esophageal wall on (*A, F*) axial T2 WI-weighted image, (*B, G*) dynamic contrast enhanced study, (*C, H*) diffusion-weighted imaging, and (*D, I*) corresponding ADC map. The ADC of the lesion was 1.42 (before therapy) and 1.92 (after therapy) $\times$ 10^{-3} mm^2/s. (*E, J*) Axial T2-weighted images showing perilesional lymphadenopathy (*arrowheads*) that decreased in size after therapy. Final pathology demonstrated esophageal squamocellular carcinoma (ypT2pN3; tumor regression grade according to Mandard: 3).

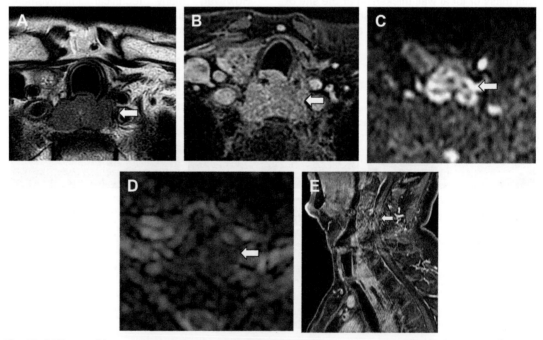

Fig. 10. A 71-year-old man with local recurrence at the anastomosis site 14 months after esophagectomy for squamocellular carcinoma of the esophagus (pT3pN0). The arrows indicate a gross anastomotic thickening on (*A*) axial T2-weighted, (*B*) dynamic contrast enhanced, (*C*) diffusion-weighted, (*D*) ADC map, and (*E*) sagittal postgadolinium T1-weighted images. The ADC value of the lesion was 0.82 $\times$ 10^{-3} mm^2/s.

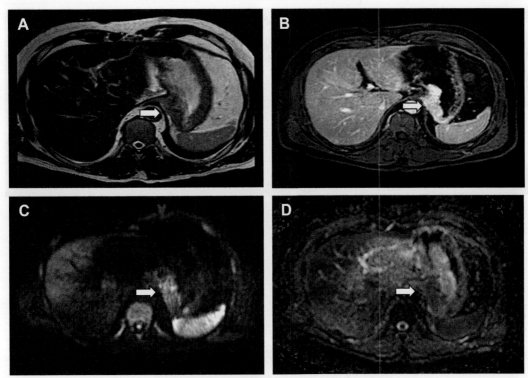

Fig. 11. Lesion involving the gastric cardia (Siewert type III) in a 52-year-old man. The arrows indicate gross thickening of the gastric wall on (A) axial T2-weighted, (B) dynamic contrast enhanced, (C) diffusion-weighted imaging, and (D) ADC map images. The ADC value of the lesion was 0.58×10^{-3} mm^2/s. Final pathology demonstrated gastric adenocarcinoma (pT3N3a).

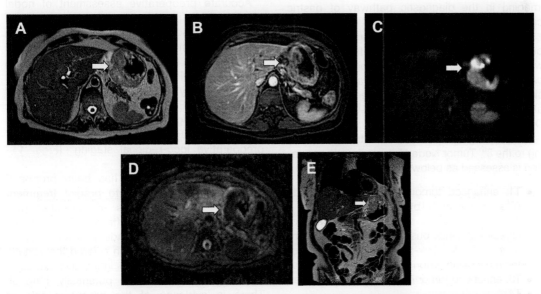

Fig. 12. Lesion involving the gastric fundus in a 76-year-old woman. The arrows indicate gross thickening of the gastric wall on (A) axial T2-weighted, (B) dynamic contrast enhanced, (C) diffusion-weighted imaging, (D) ADC map, and (E) coronal T2-weighted images. The ADC value of the lesion was 0.76×10^{-3} mm^2/s. Final pathology demonstrated gastric adenocarcinoma (pT3N3a).

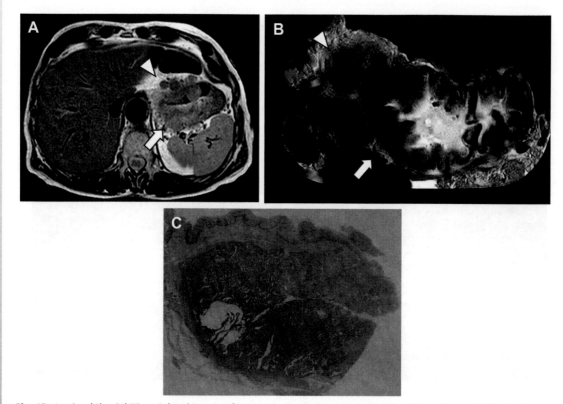

Fig. 13. In vivo (*A*) axial T2-weighted image of a gross lesion (adenocarcinoma) involving the gastric body (*arrow*) with lymphadenopathy (*arrowhead*). (*B*) T2-weighted imaging of the ex vivo specimen and (*C*) corresponding histology.

antiperistaltic agents) and also the introduction of DWI have shown the promising role of MR imaging in the diagnostic pathway of gastric cancer.

As previously mentioned, MR imaging has a high performance in depicting the different gastric wall layers. Because the detectability of gastric cancer is influenced by tumor size and local invasion, MR imaging is accurate in detecting the overall T-staging, especially when T2-WI, DWI, and DCE are combined together.[34]

On MR imaging, the depth of infiltration according to the 8th Tumor Node Metastasis[35] classification is assessed as below:

- T1: enhanced tumor that does not invade (T1a) or invades (T1b) the submucosa
- T2: continuous low-signal intensity band or enhanced cancerous portion in correspondence with the low-signal intensity band of the muscularis propria
- T3: enhanced tumor invading the subserosa
- T4
  - T4a: interrupted low-signal intensity band or enhanced cancerous portions penetrating the serosa
  - T4b: extension to the adjacent organs

Accurate preoperative assessment of nodal involvement in patients with gastric cancer is of great importance for selecting the appropriate treatment strategy. Pathologic lymph nodes have usually a short-axis diameter greater than 6 mm and regional lymph node involvement is most frequently evaluated using EUS, CT, and/or ^{18}F-FDG PET. There are as yet no robust data suggesting the superiority of MR imaging over other imaging techniques with regard to preoperative loco-regional staging[5] (**Figs. 11–13**).

However, MR imaging has been proposed as a valuable technique to predict treatment response and prognosis in selected patients.[36,37] An accurate differentiation between responders and nonresponders on MR imaging could assist the clinicians in tailored therapeutic decision making, because ineffective neoadjuvant regimens could be potentially harmful. There is evidence of the promising role of DWI and ADC of the primary tumor with regard to the response to neoadjuvant chemotherapy in gastric cancer.[5] Higher ADC values

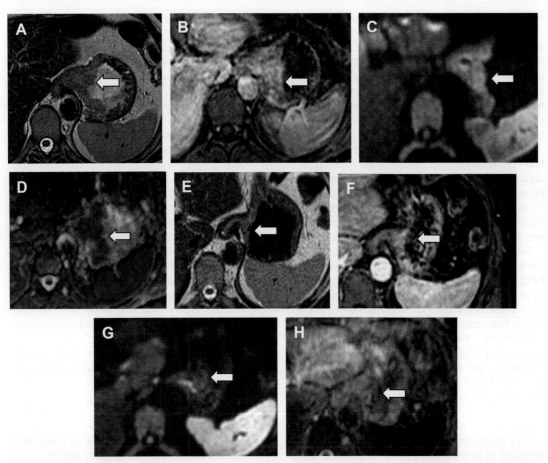

Fig. 14. Adenocarcinoma of the gastric cardia (Siewert II) in a 48-year-old man (*A–D*) before and (*E–H*) after neoadjuvant chemotherapy. The arrows indicate the lesion on (*A, E*) axial T2-WI-weighted image, (*B, F*) dynamic contrast-enhanced study, (*C, G*) diffusion-weighted imaging, and (*D, H*) corresponding ADC map. The ADC of the lesion was 1.15 (before therapy) and 2.75 (after therapy) $\times$ 10^{-3} mm^2/s. Final pathology demonstrated complete response (ypT0pN0; tumor regression grade according to Mandard: 1).

have been found in responders compared with nonresponders after neoadjuvant treatment owing to the presence of necrosis after successful treatment (ie, an increase in water diffusivity and, consequently, in ADC values)[38] (Fig. 14).

SUMMARY

MR imaging of the gastroesophageal tract has made huge advances following the technical developments and protocol optimizations that have occurred over the last decade. The new technical developments have facilitated the acquisition of high-quality multiplanar images, as well as permitting tissue characterization by means of DWI and fat suppression techniques. Despite this, several challenges still lie ahead.

There is an unmet need for standardization of MR imaging protocols, because varied studies in the gastroesophageal tract have been performed both on 1.5 T or 3 T scanners and this makes the comparison of results difficult. The lack of consensus on specific imaging sequence parameters is a great limitation, especially for quantitative image analysis. The use of different *b* values in DWI, for example, affects ADC calculation and, therefore, comparing the results from various centers and scanners is challenging. Moreover, there is no consensus on how to calculate and interpret ADC values, owing to the diverse approaches for the delineation of the regions of interest and the analysis of different ADC values (minimum, mean, or median). Similarly, there is variation for T2-WI (eg, different echo times) and DCE imaging, in which the variation for image acquisition (eg, temporal resolution) is even greater.

It follows that comparison of results across studies is difficult, and this underlines the need for a careful review of the quality of MR scanners and the reproducibility of measurement across centers, with a need to establish adequate MR imaging standards.

However, although there is still room for improvement, especially with regard to staging, evaluation of treatment response, and prognosis for esophageal and gastric cancer, the application of MR imaging in the gastroesophageal tract has a bright future.

There is also an increasing interest in the application of radiomics in esophageal and gastric cancer.[39] In the future, we can expect to see increased use of quantitative MR imaging protocols for esophageal and gastric cancers, including more robust data on ADC and other imaging biomarkers, and also from different imaging modalities.[22]

Treatment response assessment might benefit from imaging biomarkers derived from functional MR imaging, and this will certainly lead to more reproducible results and will pave to the way to the application of artificial intelligence for image interpretation.

Moreover, the integration of MR imaging findings with data from other disciplines, such as genomics and pathology, can further enhance the potential of MR imaging in the management of esophageal and gastric diseases.

In conclusion, MR imaging is a robust imaging technique for the gastrointestinal tract and its role in gastroesophageal tract is promising. The absence of ionizing radiation is important, especially for patients allergic to iodinated contrast agents and in cases of multiple follow-up studies (eg, before, during, and after therapy), where results from DWI are very promising.

However, results from large, multicentric studies are still needed to include the use of MR imaging of the gastroesophageal tract in common clinical practice.

REFERENCES

1. Sohn KM, Lee JM, Lee SY, et al. Comparing MR imaging and CT in the staging of gastric carcinoma. AJR Am J Roentgenol 2000;174(6):1551–7.
2. Hallinan JTPD, Venkatesh SK. Gastric carcinoma: imaging diagnosis, staging and assessment of treatment response. Cancer Imaging 2013;13(2):212–27.
3. Giganti F, Orsenigo E, Arcidiacono PG, et al. Preoperative locoregional staging of gastric cancer: is there a place for magnetic resonance imaging? Prospective comparison with EUS and multidetector computed tomography. Gastric Cancer 2016;19(1):216–25.
4. Borggreve AS. Imaging strategies in the management of gastric cancer: current role and future potential of MRI. Br J Radiol 2019;92(1097). 201810442019.
5. De Cobelli F, Giganti F, Orsenigo E, et al. Apparent diffusion coefficient modifications in assessing gastro-oesophageal cancer response to neoadjuvant treatment: comparison with tumour regression grade at histology. Eur Radiol 2013; 23(8):2165–74.
6. Giganti F, Salerno A, Ambrosi A, et al. Prognostic utility of diffusion-weighted MRI in oesophageal cancer: is apparent diffusion coefficient a potential marker of tumour aggressiveness? Radiol Med 2016;121(3):173–80.
7. Tofts PS, Brix G, Buckley DL, et al. Estimating kinetic parameters from dynamic contrast-enhanced T1-weighted MRI of a diffusable tracer: standardized quantities and symbols. J Magn Reson Imaging 1999;10:223–32.
8. Riddell AM, Allum WH, Thompson JN, et al. The appearances of oesophageal carcinoma demonstrated on high-resolution, T2-weighted MRI, with histopathological correlation. Eur Radiol 2007;17(2):391–9.
9. King DM, Brown G, Cunningham D, et al. Potential of surface-coil MRI for staging of esophageal cancer. AJR Am J Roentgenol 2006;187(5):1280–7.
10. Yamada I, Miyasaka N, Hikishima K, et al. Ultra-high-resolution MR imaging of esophageal carcinoma at ultra-high field strength (7.0T) ex vivo: correlation with histopathologic findings. Magn Reson Imaging 2015;33(4):413–9.
11. Kim IY, Kim SW, Shin HC, et al. MRI of gastric carcinoma: results of T and N-staging in an in vitro study. World J Gastroenterol 2009;15(32):3992–8.
12. Kang BC, Kim JH, Kim KW, et al. Abdominal imaging value of the dynamic and delayed MR sequence with Gd-DTPA in the T-staging of stomach cancer: correlation with the histopathology. Abdom Imaging 2000;25:14–24.
13. Naganawa S, Ishigaki T, Miura S, et al. MR imaging of gastric cancer in vitro: accuracy of invasion depth diagnosis. Eur Radiol 2004;14(9):1543–9.
14. Yamada I, Miyasaka N, Hikishima K, et al. Gastric carcinoma: ex vivo MR. Radiology 2015;275(3):841–8.
15. Yamada I, Saito N, Takeshita K, et al. Early gastric carcinoma: evaluation with MR imaging in vitro. Radiology 2001;220(1):115–21.
16. Jang KM, Lee KS, Lee SJ, et al. The spectrum of benign esophageal lesions: imaging findings. Korean J Radiol 2002;3(3):199–210.
17. Tsai SJ, Lin CC, Chang CW, et al. Benign esophageal lesions: endoscopic and pathologic features. World J Gastroenterol 2015;21(4):1091–8.
18. Yang PS, Lee SJ, Kim K, et al. Esophageal leiomyoma: radiologic findings in 12 patients. Korean J Radiol 2001;2(3):132–7.
19. Winant AJ, Gollub MJ, Shia J, et al. Imaging and clinicopathologic features of esophageal gastrointestinal stromal tumors. Am J Roentgenol 2014; 203(2):306–14.

20. Tomita H, Miyakawa K, Wada S, et al. The imaging features of protruding esophageal lesions. Jpn J Radiol 2016;34(5):321–30.

21. Regge D, Lo Bello G, Martincich L, et al. A case of bleeding gastric lipoma: US, CT and MR findings. Eur Radiol 1999;9(2):256–8.

22. Chagarlamudi K, Devita R, Barr RG. Gastric lipoma: a review of the literature. Ultrasound Q 2018;34(3):119–21.

23. Yu MH, Lee JM, Baek JH, et al. MRI features of gastrointestinal stromal tumors. Am J Roentgenol 2014;203(5):980–91.

24. Kang HC, Menias CO, Gaballah AH, et al. Beyond the GIST: mesenchymal tumors of the stomach. Radiographics 2013;33(6):1673–90.

25. Fitzmaurice C, Dicker D, Pain A, et al. The global burden of cancer 2013. JAMA Oncol 2015;1(4):505–27.

26. Giganti F, Ambrosi A, Petrone MC, et al. Prospective comparison of MR with diffusion-weighted imaging, endoscopic ultrasound, MDCT and positron emission tomography-CT in the pre-operative staging of oesophageal cancer: results from a pilot study. Br J Radiol 2016;89:20160087.

27. Zhu Y, Fu L, Jing W, et al. The value of magnetic resonance imaging in esophageal carcinoma: Tool or toy? Asia Pac J Clin Oncol 2019;15:101–7.

28. Lewis RB, Mehrotra AK, Rodriguez P, et al. Esophageal neoplasms: radiologic-pathologic correlation. Radiographics 2013;33:1083–108.

29. Van Rossum PSN, Van Hillegersberg R, Lever FM, et al. Imaging strategies in the management of oesophageal cancer: what's the role of MRI? Eur Radiol 2013;23(7):1753–65.

30. Heethuis SE, Goense L, van Rossum PSN, et al. DW-MRI and DCE-MRI are of complementary value in predicting pathologic response to neoadjuvant chemoradiotherapy for esophageal cancer. Acta Oncol (Madr) 2018;57(9):1201–8.

31. Knight WRC, Zylstra J, Van Hemelrijck M, et al. Patterns of recurrence in oesophageal cancer following oesophagectomy in the era of neoadjuvant chemotherapy. BJS Open 2018;1(6):182–90.

32. Kantarci M, Polat P, Alper F, et al. Comparison of CT and MRI for the diagnosis recurrent esophageal carcinoma after operation. Dis Esophagus 2004;17(1):32–7.

33. Jemal A, Bray F, Ferlay J. Global Cancer Statistics: 2011. CA Cancer J Clin 1999;49(2):1, 33–64.

34. Liu S, He J, Guan W, et al. Added value of diffusion-weighted MR imaging to T2-weighted and dynamic contrast-enhanced MR imaging in T staging of gastric cancer. Clin Imaging 2014;38(2):122–8.

35. In H, Solsky I, Palis B, et al. Validation of the 8th edition of the AJCC TNM staging system for gastric cancer using the national cancer database. Ann Surg Oncol 2017;24(12):3683–91.

36. Giganti F, Ambrosi A, Chiari D, et al. Apparent diffusion coefficient by diffusion-weighted magnetic resonance imaging as a sole biomarker for staging and prognosis of gastric cancer. Chin J Cancer Res 2017;29(2):118–26.

37. Zhong J, Zhao W, Ma W, et al. DWI as a quantitative biomarker in predicting chemotherapeutic efficacy at multitime points on gastric cancer lymph nodes metastases. Medicine (Baltimore) 2016;95(13):e3236.

38. Giganti F, Tang L, Baba H. Gastric cancer and imaging biomarkers: part 1—a critical review of DW-MRI and CE-MDCT findings. Eur Radiol 2018;29:1743–53.

39. Sah B-R, Owczarczyk K, Siddique M, et al. Radiomics in esophageal and gastric cancer. Abdom Radiol (NY) 2019;44(6):2048–58.

Magnetic Resonance of the Small Bowel: How to Do It

Darren Boone, MB BS, BSc, MD, MRCP, FRCR[a], Stuart A. Taylor, MB BS, BSc, MD, MRCP, FRCR[b,*]

KEYWORDS

- Enterography • Small bowel • MR imaging • Technique • Protocol • Preparation • Guideline

KEY POINTS

- Small bowel magnetic resonance (MR) imaging has been used in routine practice for nearly 2 decades.
- Implemented protocols still vary in patient preparation, enteric contrast, and MR imaging acquisition sequences, resulting in heterogeneous diagnostic quality.
- Consensus statements from the United States and Europe have recently been published to inform evidence-based small bowel MR imaging technique.

INTRODUCTION

Dedicated small bowel evaluation with magnetic resonance (MR) imaging has been in routine use for nearly 2 decades.[1] Once MR imaging technology advanced sufficiently to enable rapid acquisition of abdominopelvic sequences minimizing motion artifacts from peristalsis and respiration, it naturally followed that dedicated protocols to interrogate the small bowel would be performed following enteric distention with contrast medium, either administered orally (enterography) or via a nasoenteric tube (enteroclysis). As the technique evolved, many units adapted their existing abdominal imaging protocols for small bowel MR imaging, using differing bowel preparations and acquisition parameters. Consequently, heterogeneity developed in terms of institutional protocols with resulting variability in the diagnostic quality of the studies obtained. However, well-researched consensus statements have recently emerged from North America[2] and Europe[3] providing evidence-based guidance on the optimal small bowel MR imaging technique (**Table 1**). Although a detailed description of respective methodologies is beyond the scope of this article, both groups assembled panels of expert contributors and performed systematic reviews of the available literature to develop a comprehensive set of consensus recommendations. Therefore, this article presents the available research relating to the optimum small bowel MR imaging technique, summarizes the relevant US and European consensus guidance, and shares experience from the authors' daily practice.

GENERAL PATIENT PREPARATION AND BASIC MAGNETIC RESONANCE IMAGING TECHNIQUE

The aim of pretest preparation is to achieve maximal small bowel distension with enteric contrast medium while minimizing the artifacts that result from peristalsis or excessive luminal gas through use of spasmolysis and fasting.

Disclosures: D. Boone has no relationship, financial or otherwise, with a commercial company that has a direct financial interest in the subject matter or materials discussed in this article or with a company making a competing product. S.A. Taylor is a research consultant to Robarts and holds stock in Motilent.
a Department of Specialist Imaging, University College London Hospital, Podium 2, 235 Euston Road, London NW12BU, UK; b Centre for Medical Imaging, University College London, Charles Bell House, 43–45 Foley Street, London W1W 7TS, UK
* Corresponding author.
E-mail address: stuart.taylor@ucl.ac.uk

Magn Reson Imaging Clin N Am 28 (2020) 17–30
https://doi.org/10.1016/j.mric.2019.08.002

Table 1 Summary of international consensus guidance	
Patient Preparation and Basic Technique	
Patient preparation: general	Routine medications should not be stopped (V) Patients should not eat any solid food for 4–6 h (V) Patients should not drink fluids for 4–6 h except nonsparkling water (V)
Technique: enterography	There is no single preferred contrast agent for MR enterography Recommended agents include mannitol, PEG, sorbitol, and lactulose (III) The optimal volume of oral contrast is 1000–1500 mL (III) Ingestion time should be 45–60 min (V) except when previous small bowel resection If there is a stoma, it should be plugged before oral contrast ingestion (V) Laxative bowel preparation is not recommended (V) Water enema or prolonged oral contrast preparation is suggested for dedicated colonic evaluation The volume of a water for rectal enema should be based on patient tolerance
Technique: MR enteroclysis	There is no single preferred contrast agent for MR enteroclysis. Recommended agents as above Fluoroscopic guidance for NJ tube insertion before enteroclysis is mandatory (V) The NJ tube should be 8–10 F (V) Enteric contrast infusion should be via an automated pump (V) The rate of contrast infusion before MR enteroclysis should be between 80 and 120 mL/min (V) MR imaging fluoroscopic monitoring of small bowel filling during MR enteroclysis is mandatory (V) Enteric contrast progression should be monitored on the MR imaging table during MR enteroclysis (V) The optimal volume of enteric contrast should be based on real-time monitoring (V)
MR Enterography/Enteroclysis Technical Considerations and Sequence Selection	
Hardware	Both 1.5 and 3 T are adequate field strengths (II) The use of phased-array coils is mandatory (V)
Spasmolytic agents	Spasmolytic agents are recommended (II) Timing of administration should account for motion-sensitive sequences (V) The recommended first-line spasmolytic agent in Europe is 20 mg IV hyoscine butylbromide (V) The recommended second-line agent is 1 mg IV glucagon (V) (first line in United States)
Positioning	Patients can be scanned prone or supine (III)
Recommended sequences	Axial and coronal T2 FSE without FS Axial and coronal SSFPGE without FS Axial or coronal T2 FSE with FS Before and after IV contrast-enhanced 3D T1-weighted gradient-echo sequence with FS
IV contrast enhancement	In known or suspected IBD, sequences should be in the enteric (45 s) or portal venous phase (70 s) For suspected chronic GI bleeding, contrast-enhanced sequences should be in the arterial (30 s), enteric (45 s) or portal venous phase (70 s) phase IV contrast media should be pump injected with an infusion rate of 2 mL/s and a dose of 0.1–0.2 mmol/kg (V)

(Continued)	
Optional sequences	Cine motility and DWI are suggested but not mandatory (V) DWI should use a free-breathing technique (IV) DWI sequences should include b values ranging from 0 to 900 (IV) Maximal slice thickness for DWI should be 5 mm (V) Coronal diffusion-weighted sequences are not recommended (V) Dynamic contrast-enhanced sequences are suggested but not mandatory (V) Magnetization transfer sequences are not recommended (V)
Parameters	Maximal slice thickness for FSE T2W and SSFP GE sequences should be 5 mm (V) FSE T2W sequences may be performed in either 2D or 3D, although 2D is preferred (V) Maximal slice thickness for axial and coronal T1W sequences, should be 3 mm (V) T1W sequences should be performed in 3D (V)
Scan coverage and duration	Coverage should include at least the small bowel, colon, and perineum (V) Total acquisition time should be 30 min or less (V)

Final list of consensus statements (achieving agreement score of "strongly agree" or "somewhat agree" by at least 80% of panel members).

Evidence strength (Oxford Centre for Evidence-based Medicine) shown in brackets.

Abbreviations: 2D, two-dimensional; 3D, three-dimensional; DWI, diffusion-weighted imaging; FS, fat suppression; FSE, fast spin echo; GI, gastrointestinal; IBD, inflammatory bowel disease; IV, intravenous; NJ, nasojejunal; PEG, polyethylene glycol; SSFPGE, steady-state free precession gradient echo; T1W, T1 weighted; T2W, T2 weighted.

Adapted from Taylor SA, Avni F, Cronin CG, et al. The first joint ESGAR/ ESPR consensus statement on the technical performance of cross-sectional small bowel and colonic imaging. Eur Radiol 2017;27(6):2570-82.

Enteric Contrast Administration

Pretest preparation

Although many clinicians consider that fasting for 4 to 6 hours improves tolerance of oral contrast medium, there is no strong supportive evidence. Fasting for 2 to 4 hours may be sufficient.[2] Nonetheless, it is universally accepted that patients should continue their regular oral medication and avoid ingestion of carbonated drinks because of the risk of producing intraluminal gas artifacts. Clear fluids are generally thought to be acceptable; the authors find that a 4-hour solid food fast improves oral contrast ingestion and image quality while remaining well tolerated.

Enteric contrast medium

There is good evidence that the accuracy of MR imaging is improved by administration of oral contrast[4] and this is currently considered the standard of care recommended by both US[2] and European[3] consensus guidance (**Fig. 1**). Collapsed bowel can both hide and mimic small bowel disease.

Choice of contrast agent Ideal enteric contrast media should maximize luminal distension along the entire small bowel for the duration of the study. Water is generally insufficient. Hyperosmolar agents reduce gut absorption and viscous fluids tend to promote distension. Although so-called dark lumen imaging using superparamagnetic iron oxide nanoparticles (**Fig. 2**) is favored by a few centers,[5] use of media that produce characteristic luminal T2 hyperintensity to achieve maximum contrast against the bowel wall (**Fig. 3**) is now almost universal. Such agents are hypointense to the bowel wall on T1-weighted sequences such that bowel wall enhancement is readily appreciated[6–8] (**Fig. 4**). Consequently, several oral contrast agents have been tested and their resulting properties described in the literature,[5,9–13] but no strong evidence from patient cohorts supports one particular agent more than another. Nevertheless, a consistent finding is that distension is improved by hyperosmolar agents,[13,14] particularly when ingested between 45 and 60 minutes before the examination.[8]

Commonly used T2-hyperintense contrast media include polyethylene glycol (PEG) and mannitol solution in varying concentrations, often prepared locally with or without bulking agents such as locust bean or xanthan gum. In the United States, 0.1% low-density barium sulfate suspension is also commonly administered.[2] Available superparamagnetic iron oxide contrast agents are

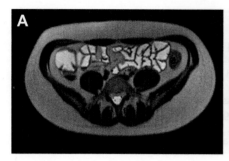
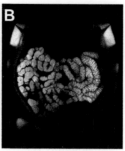

Fig. 1. Luminal distension with enteric contrast media at MR enterography. (A) Axial half Fourier acquisition single-shot turbo spin echo (HASTE) sequence obtained at 1.5 T shows distal ileal loops and cecum with well-distended ileal loops with T2-hyperintense oral contrast medium. (B) Coronal HASTE imaging at 3 T following spectral fat suppression shows optimum distension of jejunal and ileal loops.

proprietary formulations subject to local regulatory approval and much less frequently used.[5,11] The European consensus statement states that, given the lack of evidence suggesting superiority of one preparation compared with another, the decision is left to clinician preference. In our practice, the authors find a simple 2.5% mannitol solution offers reproducible signal characteristics, luminal transit, and distension without compromising patient acceptability, cost, or safety. In addition, we

have seen that refrigeration and flavoring (eg, with blackcurrant cordial) enhances compliance, particularly in children. It should be remembered that hyperosmolar agents often cause abdominal bloating and diarrhea, which are often identified by patients as the worst part of the examination.[15] Patients should therefore be appropriately counseled about such side effects and given advice on symptom management, postexamination travel, and so forth.

Contrast volume and timing

Limited evidence relates to optimal enteric contrast volume. For example, a study of 10 healthy volunteers showed that volumes of less than 1000 mL resulted in inferior distension,[12] whereas others have shown that reasonable-quality examinations can be obtained with as little as 450 mL of oral contrast media.[16] Consequently, neither US nor European panels reached consensus on the minimum acceptable enteric oral contrast volume; in clinical practice, this is usually judged on a case-by-case basis. Similarly, scant evidence exists for the optimal duration of enteric contrast ingestion and whether to split into divided doses or drink continuously. The authors aim to administer 1600 mL of 2% mannitol solution over 1 hour for routine small bowel studies and 1000 mL over 45 minutes if there has been extensive prior small bowel resection. It is imperative that the need for consumption of oral contrast is explained to patients and advice given on the methods of ingestion over the preexamination time period. In our experience, such counseling improves the quality of examinations. If an ileostomy is present, plugging is recommended by European guidance to improve enteric distension. However, there is no direct evidence to support this approach and, for pragmatic reasons, the authors do not routinely do this.

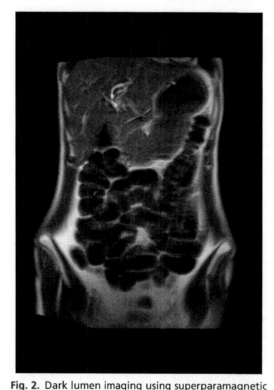

Fig. 2. Dark lumen imaging using superparamagnetic iron oxide nanoparticles. T2-weighted coronal HASTE sequence following 900 mL of oral contrast medium containing iron oxide nanoparticles enteric contrast administration. Note the intermediate-signal small bowel wall appears hyperintense relative to the homogeneous T2 hypointense luminal content. (Courtesy of F. Maccioni MD, PhD, Rome, Italy.)

Use of rectal enema

Although there is some evidence that use of rectal contrast administration may assist in

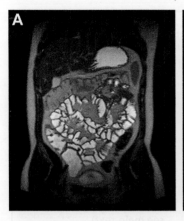
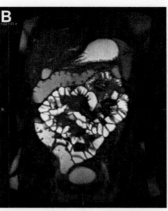

Fig. 3. Small bowel MR imaging following T2-hyperintense enteric contrast media. Coronal HASTE sequences have been obtained at 1.5 T (*A*) without and (*B*) with fat suppression at the level of the ileocecal valve. The characteristic T2-hyperintense luminal content provides optimal contrast with the adjacent bowel wall. The terminal ileum is slightly thickened with subtle loss of normal architecture, but there is no mural edema to suggest active inflammation.

demonstration of the ileocecal junction,[6] this is not recommended. Specific colonic evaluation as part of small bowel MR imaging protocols is discussed in further detail later.

Enteroclysis

Enteroclysis is designed to achieve optimal luminal distension via direct administration of enteric contrast into the jejunum via a nasojejunal tube.[17,18] Some studies have shown improved small bowel distension compared with routine oral contrast administration,[18] but a meaningful impact on clinical decision making has not been shown.[19] Furthermore, because enteroclysis requires placement of a nasoenteric feeding tube, usually under fluoroscopic control, it is invasive and hence potential improvement in technical

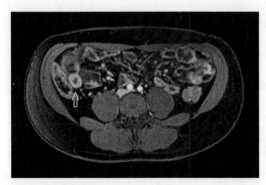

Fig. 4. T1-weighted imaging following intravenous contrast enhancement. Typical T2-hyperintense enteric contrast agents are hypointense to the bowel wall on T1-weighted sequences, enabling abnormal mural enhancement to be readily appreciated following intravenous contrast administration. Axial three-dimensional gradient-echo sequences allow acquisition of an entire abdominopelvic volume during a single breath hold. The terminal ileum (*arrow*) is hyperenhancing relative to the adjacent, normal small bowel loops.

quality must be weighed against impact on compliance and radiation exposure.

The optimal volume of enteric contrast for MR enteroclysis should be based on real-time monitoring; delivery via an automated pump system is preferred but not mandatory. In all other respects, international guidance essentially mirrors that of MR enterography for patient preparation, positioning, and acquisition protocol. Overall, although acknowledging this technique can be valuable (eg, to show adhesions or luminal filling defects such as polyps), enteroclysis is not considered necessary for effective small bowel MR imaging in inflammatory bowel disease by either US or European consensus guidance.

TECHNICAL CONSIDERATIONS AND SEQUENCE SELECTION
Patient Positioning

Although some data suggest superior luminal distension can be achieved when prone,[20] and that prone positioning may decrease coronal sequence acquisition time by compressing the abdomen, there is no hard evidence that this improves diagnostic accuracy.[20] Moreover, some patients find this position difficult, particularly those with a stoma, hence supine positioning is also considered acceptable. In our practice, the authors attempt prone imaging wherever possible because we observer fewer respiratory motion artifacts and improved acceptability for those who find MR imaging claustrophobic.

Spasmolysis

Although some studies have suggested that satisfactory small bowel MR imaging can be achieved without the use of a spasmolytic,[21] many show significantly superior distension with the use of these agents,[22] particularly proximally. Furthermore, reduction in peristalsis-related motion artifact improves study quality. International guidance therefore recommends spasmolysis before MR enterography. The evidence suggests that both glucagon and hyoscine butylbromide are acceptable, albeit with differing onset and duration of effect. Both are most effective when given intravenously.[23]

Although data from healthy volunteers suggests that glucagon is superior to hyoscine butylbromide for achieving complete aperistalsis,[24] there is currently no evidence that this improves diagnostic accuracy. Therefore, based on expert opinion, cost, and availability, in Europe, 20 mg of hyoscine butylbromide is recommended as the first-line spasmolytic, with 1 mg of glucagon as second line. Either a single or a split dose is acceptable. In the United States, where regulatory approval differs, intravenous (IV) glucagon is considered first line.[25] Because of the short half-life, spasmolytics should be administered directly before motion-sensitive sequences, such as T2-weighted imaging and three-dimensional (3D) T1-weighted postcontrast series (postcontrast-enhanced images are particularly sensitive to peristaltic motion artifact). Intramuscular administration can also be considered if necessary; it is longer lasting but less predictable.[23] Both EU and US guidance mandate evaluation for contraindications or drug interactions before antispasmodic and contrast administration. The authors' current MRE protocol is summarized in **Table 2**.

Magnetic Resonance Imaging Acquisition

Hardware

There is currently no EU or US consensus regarding optimal field strength for small bowel MR imaging; available evidence confirms that high-quality acquisitions are possible at both 3 T and 1.5 T.[26,27] The use of phased-array coils is recommended regardless of field strength. The authors routinely perform enterography at both field strengths, using an extralarge torso coil, with slight parameter modifications as detailed in **Tables 3** and **4**.

Essential sequences

Basic considerations As with routine abdomino-pelvic studies, multiplanar imaging is recommended. Coronal plane imaging, in addition to routine axial sequences, is considered essential to small bowel MR imaging; it is mandated by European and US guidance. Suggested maximal slice thicknesses are 5 mm for T2-weighted imaging and 3 mm for 3D T1-weighted sequences. Both European and US guidelines currently recommend a basic set of acquisition sequences (balanced steady-state free precession gradient-echo

Table 2 Example patient preparation protocol from the authors' institution	
Patient Preparation	Continue routine medications No solid food for 4 h; nonsparkling water only for 4 h Patient arrives 1 h before scan Enteric contrast; 1600 mL of 2% mannitol over 40 min (or 2500 mL in 2 divided doses over 3 h in specific cases in which dedicated colonic imaging is indicated; see main text) Patient consent and suitability for IV spasmolytic and IV gadolinium contrast enhancement confirmed (if indicated) Patients positioned prone with arms above head if possible; feet first if claustrophobic
Scanning Technique	1.5-T or 3-T platform with large torso phased-array coils Scan coverage is from diaphragm to perineum; if detailed perineal imaging is required, additional fistula protocol Total acquisition time is just <30 min
Sequences	Sequences acquired as per **Table 3** (1.5 T, Siemens Avanto) and **Table 4** (3T Philips Achieva) Additional sagittal cine sequences if adhesions are suspected IV gadolinium administration only in known/suspected penetrating disease. If administered, pump injection of 2 mL/s infusion rate, dose of 0.1 mmol/kg and images acquired at 70 s

[SSFPGR], T2-weighted images [with and without fat saturation], and T1-weighted sequences before and after gadolinium enhancement), together with useful but optional sequences (notably diffusion-weighted imaging [DWI] and cine motility).

T2-weighted imaging T2-weighted imaging (with and without fat suppression) is considered the cornerstone of small bowel MR imaging, in

Table 3
Example small bowel magnetic resonance imaging protocol for 1.5 T (Siemens Avanto)

Step	Sequence	Plane	2D/3D	ST (mm)	TR	TE	FS
1	Localizer						
2	T2 TRUFI coronal BH 4 mm	Cor	2D	4	3.45	1.46	No
3	T2 TRUFI transverse BH 4 mm	Ax	2D	4	3.73	1.87	No
4	T2 TRUFI coronal BH 20 measures (motility study)	Cor	2D	10	3.57	1.79	No
5	Hyoscine Butylbromide 10 mg						
6	T2 HASTE coronal BH 4 mm	Cor	2D	4	600	87	No
7	T2 HASTE coronal BH 4 mm FS	Cor	2D	4	500	87	Yes
8	T2 HASTE transverse BH 4 mm	Ax	2D	4	500	87	No
9	T2 HASTE transverse BH 4 mm FS	Ax	2D	4	500	87	Yes
10	DWI ep2d diff 3av (b values 0, 600; 3 averages)	Ax	2D	5	2500	85	Yes
11	Hyoscine Butylbromide 10 mg if IV Contrast Indicated						
12	T1 VIBE coronal BH FS precontrast	Ax	3D	3.5	3.24	1.1	Yes
13	IV Gd Contrast Administration						
14	T1 VIBE coronal FS BH postcontrast	Cor	3D	3.5	3.24	1.1	Yes
15	T1 VIBE FS transverse BH postcontrast	Ax	3D	3	4.89	2.39	Yes

Abbreviations: Ax, axial; Cor, coronal; BH, breath hold; DWI ep2d diff 3 av, diffusion weighted imaging, echo planar imaging 2d multislice diffusion imaging, 3 averages; FS, fat saturation; HASTE, half Fourier acquisition single-shot turbo spin echo; ST, slice thickness; TE, echo time; TR, repetition time; TRUFI, true fast imaging with steady-state free precession; VIBE, volumetric interpolated breath-hold examination.

Table 4
Example small bowel magnetic resonance imaging protocol for 3T (Philips Achieva)

Step No	Sequence	Plane	2D/3D	ST (mm)	TR	TE	FS
1	Localizer						
2	BTFE BH coronal	Cor	2D	5	2.6	1.32	No
3	BTFE 5 mm coronal: 30 measures (motility study)	Cor	2D	5	3.7	1.85	No
4	Hyoscine Butylbromide 10 mg						
5	HASTE BH transverse	Ax	2D	5	1100	80	No
6	HASTE BH coronal	Cor	2D	4	1200	80	No
7	T2 FS BH transverse	Ax	2D	7	1450	70	Yes
8	T2 FS BH coronal	Cor	2D	7	1882	70	Yes
9	BFFE BH transverse	Ax	2D	7	1450	70	No
10	DWI transverse (b values, 0, 50, 600)	Ax	2D	4	2.3	1.13	Yes
11	Hyoscine Butylbromide 10 mg if IV Contrast Indicated						
12	THRIVE precontrast coronal	Cor	3D	4	2.3	1.13	Yes
13	IV Gd contrast administration						
14	THRIVE postcontrast coronal	Cor	3D	4	2.3	1.13	Yes
15	THRIVE postcontrast transverse	Ax	3D	4	2.2	1.09	Yes

Abbreviations: BFFE, balanced fast-field echo; BTFE, balanced turbo-field echo; THRIVE, T1 high-resolution isotropic volume excitation.

particular to evaluate active inflammation. Identifying mural edema is fundamental to assessing disease activity and is best judged on fluid-sensitive T2-weighted sequences (**Fig. 5**). Homogeneous fat suppression may be accomplished by various techniques, including chemically selective fat saturation, Dixon-based methods, short tau inversion recovery, and spectral adiabatic inversion recovery,[28,29] although not all methods lend themselves to the rapid sequence acquisition times required for abdominopelvic imaging. Similarly, because peristalsis-mediated artifacts are not mitigated by breath-holding or respiratory triggering techniques, motion-insensitive single-shot techniques are considered the most reliable. There is no available evidence regarding the optimal combination of regular fast spin echo T2-weighted and SSFPGR sequences, with many published studies using both. SSFPGR sequences are relatively insensitive to motion artifacts and provide clear definition of the bowel wall and mesenteric structures such as vessels and lymph nodes; the authors use them routinely in our practice. They are also frequently used in cine motility imaging (discussed later).

T1-weighted sequences Gradient-echo (GRE) and fast spin echo techniques can be used to obtain

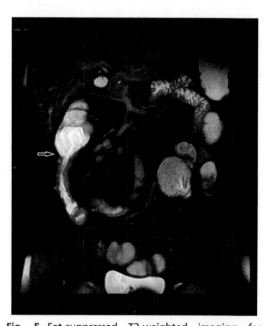

Fig. 5. Fat-suppressed T2-weighted imaging for showing active mural inflammation. Fat-suppressed coronal HASTE imaging acquired at 3 T through the ileocolonic anastomosis (*arrow*) shows florid T2-hyperintense submucosal edema, luminal narrowing, and loss of architecture involving a long segment of actively inflamed neoterminal ileum.

T1-weighted small bowel MR imaging. Three-dimensional GRE sequences have the advantage of rapid acquisition times that enable imaging within the duration of 1 breath hold for most patients. This technique minimizes respiratory motion artifact, allows dynamic contrast enhancement via rapid repeated acquisitions, and is recommended by current US guidance. However, recent developments in vendor technology, such as radial 3D GRE sequences, allow free-breathing T1-weighted imaging, which shows promise for patients who cannot breath hold.[30,31] European guidance does not specify T1 parameters; the authors perform 3D spoiled GRE acquisitions.

Intravenous contrast enhancement

IV gadolinium contrast enhancement is important for comprehensive abdominopelvic MR imaging, particularly for abscesses, collections, and fistulae. Furthermore, postcontrast images are considered valuable for showing mural inflammation, fibrosis,[32–34] and loop tethering.[35] Research suggests that use of postgadolinium T1-weighted images increases diagnostic accuracy,[36,37] and bowel wall enhancement is a component of some validated disease activity scores.[38,39] Consequently, IV contrast is currently recommended by both European and US consensus guidelines, with the latter stating that every attempt should be made to administer unless contraindicated; for example, by allergy or pregnancy. The optimal timing of sequences acquisition after injection can either be in the enteric or portal venous phase (45–70 seconds).

However, in our practice, the authors are becoming cautious regarding using IV contrast media in view of the increasing evidence of possible neuronal retention of gadolinium.[40] This possibility is of particular concern because of the generally young age of the imaged patient population and the need for frequent repeat imaging in those with inflammatory bowel disease (IBD). Moreover, in our experience, DWI can often provide equivalent information, albeit with a steep learning curve. There is increasing evidence that diagnostic accuracy can be maintained even if gadolinium administration is omitted, particularly if DWI is performed[41,42] (discussed later). Furthermore, validated MR disease activity scores do not always require assessment of postgadolinium-enhanced images.[43,44] Based on this emerging evidence, and our own 15-year experience of interpreting MR enterography, in our practice we no longer perform IV contrast enhancement in routine outpatient examinations, relying on T2-weighted sequences, DWI, and cine motility sequences

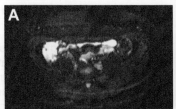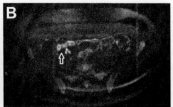

Fig. 6. DWI. Increasing evidence supports the role of DWI for identification and quantification of inflammation. In this example, axial DWI obtained at 1.5 T with b values of (*A*) 0 and (*B*) 600 shows subtle restricted diffusion involving 6 cm of terminal ileum (*arrow*). The highest b value should be chosen such that the normal bowel wall should be barely conspicuous to maximize contrast with hyperintense mural disorder.

alone. However, we usually administer IV gadolinium for known penetrating disease, particularly if there is a suggestion of abscess or fistula.

Diffusion-weighted imaging

Although considered optional by both European and US guidelines, the use of DWI is increasingly established in small bowel MR imaging protocols in many institutions, with evidence supporting its role for identification and quantification of inflammation,[45–50] and as a potential replacement for IV contrast-enhanced sequences.[51] Improvement in diagnostic utility compared with conventional MR imaging sequences is yet to be fully established,[52] in part explaining why it is considered optional at present by the European and US expert panels. Furthermore, specificity is at best moderate,[52] with collapsed bowel and lymphoid hyperplasia frequent causes of false-positive findings. If used, DWI sequences must be interpreted alongside conventional sequences to avoid misdiagnosis. Nonetheless, it is widely acknowledged that DWI may have a particular place in pediatric imaging[53]; specific recommendations are provided later. Locally, the authors perform DWI on all patients as part of our routine protocol using b values of 0, 50, and 600 s/mm². European guidelines suggested that, if performed, DWI should be acquired in the axial plane, during free breathing, with a maximal slice thickness of 5 mm³ (**Fig. 6**).

Motility/cine sequences

Dynamic small bowel motility MR imaging can be achieved by performing rapid repeated slices through a single slice or region of interest,[54–56] typically using SSFPGR-based sequences and usually using a slice thickness of around 6 to 10 mm (**Fig. 7**). The concept is to capture real-time bowel peristalsis at high temporal resolution and, although acquisitions can be targeted (eg, on an inflamed terminal ileum), usually data are acquired from the whole small bowel volume by sequential repeated coronal acquisitions in differing anatomic locations. Small bowel affected by IBD shows altered motility, with reduction correlated to underlying inflammatory activity.[57] Increasing evidence suggest that cine imaging can improve diagnostic accuracy,[58,59] aid evaluation of disease activity,[57,60–62] and evaluate response to treatment.[63] However, both European and US recommendations currently consider cine motility MR imaging as optional. In our practice, we find cine motility imaging is useful to assess the severity of inflammation and subsequent treatment response, as well as local and upstream bowel function in apparent strictures. We acquire multiple coronal thick-slab cine images for all patients, with the addition of deep breathing sagittal motility sequences if abdominal wall adhesions are suspected.

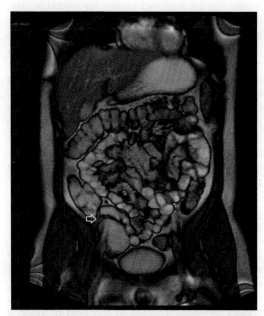

Fig. 7. Dynamic small bowel motility MR imaging. Real-time cine imaging can be achieved by performing rapid repeated acquisitions through a single slice, typically using an SSFPGR sequence with a slice thickness of 6 to 10 mm. For example, this coronal TRUFI (true fast imaging with steady-state free precession) sequence at the level of the ileocecal valve (*arrow*) can enable evaluation of terminal ileal peristalsis.

Magnetization transfer and T2*

Magnetization transfer[64] and T2*[65] sequences are promising for quantification of fibrosis, but, although supportive data are slowly emerging, they are as yet insufficient to recommend use outside a research setting. The authors do not currently perform these sequences in our routine practice.

PEDIATRIC PATIENTS: SPECIFIC CONSIDERATIONS

Although the pediatric small bowel MR imaging technique tends to mirror that of adults,[66,67] there are important exceptions. Children are less likely to tolerate prolonged fasting or fluid restriction and, according to expert opinion, the duration should be based on the child's age in line with local practice. Similarly, doses of enteric contrast, IV gadolinium, and spasmolysis vary compared with the adult population and should be calculated based on the child's weight using locally agreed formulae.

Although there are data supporting the benefits of glucagon on image quality, glucagon results in nausea for around half of pediatric patients.[25,68] Furthermore, administration prolongs scan duration, requires cannulation, and it may not be licensed locally for pediatric use. Moreover, high diagnostic accuracy can also be achieved without spasmolysis[69] and hence spasmolytic use is considered optional by consensus opinion.

Although IV gadolinium remains recommended in the pediatric age group, alternative techniques, including DWI and motility imaging, are current research priorities because of increasing concerns surrounding some gadolinium contrast agents.[40] In general, MR imaging technique and sequence parameters align with adult practice.

BEYOND THE SMALL BOWEL: COLONIC AND EXTRALUMINAL IMAGING

Small bowel MR imaging inevitably images the extraluminal solid viscera and colon, but the extent varies according to acquisition technique. For example, although the perianal tissues should be encompassed in the field of view, it is neither practical nor appropriate to perform dedicated high-resolution fistula sequences in all cases. Likewise, although it is often possible to show active colitis following small bowel preparation, modifications to routine technique are required if more detailed colonic imaging is required.

Colonic Preparation for Small Bowel Magnetic Resonance Imaging

Although routine use of laxatives is not recommended, there is good evidence that detection of colitis is improved with administration of a water enema after bowel preparation compared with evaluating the unprepared colon during small bowel MR imaging.[6,70–72] An alternative approach to improve colonic evaluation is prolonged oral preparation.[7] In our practice, for individual cases in which colonic evaluation is required, we use the VIGOR++ (VIrtual GastrOintestinal tRact) study protocol,[73] comprising a total of 2400 mL of 2.5% mannitol solution, in 2 doses: 800 mL 3 hours before the examination and 1600 mL 1 hour pretest to achieve distension of both colonic and small bowel segments. This method gives excellent distension of both large and small bowel loops but at the expense of patient experience, because of the increased volume of oral contrast and subsequent gastrointestinal side effects (**Fig. 8**). Nonetheless, sensitivity for early mucosal disease remains low.[74]

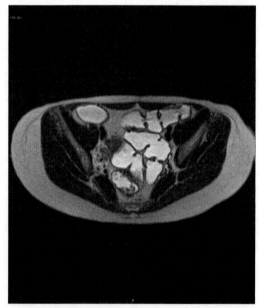

Fig. 8. Modified technique for colonic imaging with MR enterography. When dedicated colonic evaluation is required, the authors perform prolonged oral contrast administration in accordance with the VIGOR++ study protocol (see text). This method gives excellent distension of both large and small bowel loops, but at the expense of patient experience because of the additional contrast volume and ingestion duration. In this example, contrast has reached the rectum; the sigmoid is well distended and the wall is well shown.

Extraluminal Assessment

A comprehensive small bowel MR imaging protocol typically involves multiplanar multiparametric sequences including IV contrast enhancement and DWI. Therefore, it can be used to simultaneously evaluate the extraluminal structures. However, routine protocols are optimized to image the small bowel within an acceptable time frame, and consequently neither the coverage nor the resolution through surrounding structures is likely sufficient for detailed assessment. For example, the cranial aspects of the liver and spleen are often excluded from the field of view to reduce the duration of breath-hold sequences and DWI may be targeted; for example, to the ileocecal junction. Therefore, although some solid organ disorders can be shown well, this can be considered serendipitous rather than an inevitable advantage of the technique. Little overlap exists between small bowel MR imaging and other imaging protocols, such as magnetic resonance cholangiopancreatography, and, in our experience, it is often more appropriate to perform dedicated studies on a separate occasion, unless MR imaging is performed under sedation or general anesthesia. The key consideration is to communicate the limitations of the technique to the referring clinician or to recommend additional focused sequences if appropriate.

SUMMARY

Although recent European and Northern American consensus statements have been developed from comprehensive literature reviews and expert opinion, small bowel MR imaging technique remains variable in daily practice and there is a need for continued research to expand the evidence base.

In summary, small bowel MR imaging should be performed following enteric contrast administration, usually ingested orally, or in specific circumstances via a fluoroscopically positioned nasojejunal tube. Several media are acceptable, but hyperosmolar, viscous liquid with a hyperintense T2 and hypointense T1 signal is almost universally favored. Volumes vary, but for routine adult examinations a minimum of 1 L should be given over at least 45 minutes. IV spasmolysis should be administered unless contraindicated, preferably just before motion-sensitive sequences, and 3-T and 1.5-T machines with phased-array coils are acceptable. T2-weighted sequences with and without fat suppression are the cornerstone of imaging; axial and coronal planes are advised. IV contrast enhancement is currently recommended, although increasingly some institutions (including the authors') are omitting this in outpatient follow-up examinations, particularly if they have local expertise with DWI and cine motility imaging. Although DWI and cine sequences are currently considered optional, the evidence base for their use continues to grow and many centers implement 1 or both of these sequences routinely. Although small bowel MR imaging includes the colon and solid viscera, the examination is optimized for the small intestine and extraluminal evaluation is often limited; good communication with referring clinicians is essential to ensure appropriate expectations from the examination.

REFERENCES

1. Lomas DJ, Graves MJ. Small bowel MRI using water as a contrast medium. Br J Radiol 1999;72(862): 994–7.
2. Grand DJ, Guglielmo FF, Al-Hawary MM. MR enterography in Crohn's disease: current consensus on optimal imaging technique and future advances from the SAR Crohn's disease-focused panel. Abdom Imaging 2015;40(5):953–64.
3. Taylor SA, Avni F, Cronin CG, et al. The first joint ESGAR/ESPR consensus statement on the technical performance of cross-sectional small bowel and colonic imaging. Eur Radiol 2017;27(6):2570–82.
4. Jesuratnam-Nielsen K, Løgager VB, Rezanavaz-Gheshlagh B, et al. Plain magnetic resonance imaging as an alternative in evaluating inflammation and bowel damage in inflammatory bowel disease–a prospective comparison with conventional magnetic resonance follow-through. Scand J Gastroenterol 2015;50(5):519–27.
5. Maccioni F, Viscido A, Marini M, et al. MRI evaluation of Crohn's disease of the small and large bowel with the use of negative superparamagnetic oral contrast agents. Abdom Imaging 2002;27(4):384–93.
6. Ajaj W, Lauenstein TC, Langhorst J, et al. Small bowel hydro-MR imaging for optimized ileocecal distension in Crohn's disease: should an additional rectal enema filling be performed? J Magn Reson Imaging 2005;22(1):92–100.
7. Cronin CG, Lohan DG, Browne AM, et al. Does MRI with oral contrast medium allow single-study depiction of inflammatory bowel disease enteritis and colitis? Eur Radiol 2010;20(7):1667–74.
8. Kuehle CA, Ajaj W, Ladd SC, et al. Hydro-MRI of the small bowel: effect of contrast volume, timing of contrast administration, and data acquisition on bowel distention. AJR Am J Roentgenol 2006; 187(4):W375–85.
9. Ippolito D, Invernizzi F, Galimberti S, et al. MR enterography with polyethylene glycol as oral contrast

medium in the follow-up of patients with Crohn disease: comparison with CT enterography. Abdom Imaging 2010;35(5):563–70.

10. Laghi A, Paolantonio P, Iafrate F, et al. MR of the small bowel with a biphasic oral contrast agent (polyethylene glycol): technical aspects and findings in patients affected by Crohn's disease. Radiol Med 2003;106(1–2):18–27.

11. Markova I, Polakova K, Tucek P, et al. MR enterography with a new negative oral contrast solution containing maghemite nanoparticles. Biomed Pap Med Fac Univ Palacky Olomouc Czech Repub 2012;156(3):229–35.

12. Ajaj W, Goehde SC, Schneemann H, et al. Oral contrast agents for small bowel MRI: comparison of different additives to optimize bowel distension. Eur Radiol 2004;14(3):458–64.

13. Ajaj W, Goyen M, Schneemann H, et al. Oral contrast agents for small bowel distension in MRI: influence of the osmolarity for small bowel distention. Eur Radiol 2005;15(7):1400–6.

14. Borthne AS, Abdelnoor M, Storaas T, et al. Osmolarity: a decisive parameter of bowel agents in intestinal magnetic resonance imaging. Eur Radiol 2006; 16(6):1331–6.

15. Miles A, Bhatnagar G, Halligan S, et al. Magnetic resonance enterography, small bowel ultrasound and colonoscopy to diagnose and stage Crohn's disease: patient acceptability and perceived burden. Eur Radiol 2019;29(3):1083–93.

16. Kinner S, Kuehle CA, Herbig S, et al. MRI of the small bowel: can sufficient bowel distension be achieved with small volumes of oral contrast? Eur Radiol 2008;18(11):2542–8.

17. Masselli G, Vecchioli A, Gualdi GF. Crohn disease of the small bowel: MR enteroclysis versus conventional enteroclysis. Abdom Imaging 2006;31(4): 400–9.

18. Masselli G, Casciani E, Polettini E, et al. Comparison of MR enteroclysis with MR enterography and conventional enteroclysis in patients with Crohn's disease. Eur Radiol 2008;18(3):438–47.

19. Negaard A, Paulsen V, Sandvik L, et al. A prospective randomized comparison between two MRI studies of the small bowel in Crohn's disease, the oral contrast method and MR enteroclysis. Eur Radiol 2007;17(9):2294–301.

20. Cronin CG, Lohan DG, Mhuircheartaigh JN, et al. MRI small-bowel follow-through: prone versus supine patient positioning for best small-bowel distention and lesion detection. AJR Am J Roentgenol 2008;191(2):502–6.

21. Grand DJ, Beland MD, Machan JT, et al. Detection of Crohn's disease: comparison of CT and MR enterography without anti-peristaltic agents performed on the same day. Eur J Radiol 2012;81(8):1735–41.

22. Cronin CG, Dowd G, Mhuircheartaigh JN, et al. Hypotonic MR duodenography with water ingestion alone: feasibility and technique. Eur Radiol 2009; 19(7):1731–5.

23. Gutzeit A, Binkert CA, Koh DM, et al. Evaluation of the anti-peristaltic effect of glucagon and hyoscine on the small bowel: comparison of intravenous and intramuscular drug administration. Eur Radiol 2012; 22(6):1186–94.

24. Froehlich JM, Daenzer M, von Weymarn C, et al. Aperistaltic effect of hyoscine N-butylbromide versus glucagon on the small bowel assessed by magnetic resonance imaging. Eur Radiol 2009; 19(6):1387–93.

25. Dillman JR, Smith EA, Khalatbari S, et al. I.v. glucagon use in pediatric MR enterography: effect on image quality, length of examination, and patient tolerance. AJR Am J Roentgenol 2013;201(1):185–9.

26. Fiorino G, Bonifacio C, Padrenostro M, et al. Comparison between 1.5 and 3.0 Tesla magnetic resonance enterography for the assessment of disease activity and complications in ileo-colonic Crohn's disease. Dig Dis Sci 2013;58(11):3246–55.

27. Jiang X, Asbach P, Hamm B, et al. MR imaging of distal ileal and colorectal chronic inflammatory bowel disease–diagnostic accuracy of 1.5 T and 3 T MRI compared to colonoscopy. Int J Colorectal Dis 2014;29(12):1541–50.

28. Lauenstein TC, Sharma P, Hughes T, et al. Evaluation of optimized inversion-recovery fat-suppression techniques for T2-weighted abdominal MR imaging. J Magn Reson Imaging 2008;27(6):1448–54.

29. Udayasankar UK, Martin D, Lauenstein T, et al. Role of spectral presaturation attenuated inversion-recovery fat-suppressed T2-weighted MR imaging in active inflammatory bowel disease. J Magn Reson Imaging 2008;28(5):1133–40.

30. Chandarana H, Block TK, Rosenkrantz AB, et al. Free-breathing radial 3D fat-suppressed T1-weighted gradient echo sequence: a viable alternative for contrast-enhanced liver imaging in patients unable to suspend respiration. Invest Radiol 2011; 46(10):648–53.

31. Azevedo RM, de Campos RO, Ramalho M, et al. Free-breathing 3D T1-weighted gradient-echo sequence with radial data sampling in abdominal MRI: preliminary observations. AJR Am J Roentgenol 2011;197(3):650–7.

32. Aisen AM. Science to practice: can the diagnosis of fibrosis with magnetization contrast MR aid in the evaluation of patients with Crohn disease? Radiology 2011;259(1):1–3.

33. Fallis SA, Murphy P, Sinha R, et al. Magnetic resonance enterography in Crohn's disease: a comparison with the findings at surgery. Colorectal Dis 2013;15(10):1273–80.

34. Fornasa F, Benassuti C, Benazzato L. Role of magnetic resonance enterography in differentiating between fibrotic and active inflammatory small bowel stenosis in patients with Crohn's disease. J Clin Imaging Sci 2011;1:35.

35. Ramalho M, Heredia V, Cardoso C, et al. Magnetic resonance imaging of small bowel Crohn's disease. Acta Med Port 2012;25(4):231–40.

36. Maccioni F, Bruni A, Viscido A, et al. MR imaging in patients with Crohn disease: value of T2- versus T1-weighted gadolinium-enhanced MR sequences with use of an oral superparamagnetic contrast agent. Radiology 2006;238(2):517–30.

37. Low RN, Sebrechts CP, Politoske DA, et al. Crohn disease with endoscopic correlation: single-shot fast spin-echo and gadolinium-enhanced fat-suppressed spoiled gradient-echo MR imaging. Radiology 2002;222(3):652–60.

38. Rimola J, Ordás I, Rodriguez S, et al. Magnetic resonance imaging for evaluation of Crohn's disease: validation of parameters of severity and quantitative index of activity. Inflamm Bowel Dis 2011;17(8):1759–68.

39. Makanyanga JC, Pendsé D, Dikaios N, et al. Evaluation of Crohn's disease activity: initial validation of a magnetic resonance enterography global score (MEGS) against faecal calprotectin. Eur Radiol 2014;24(2):277–87.

40. Flood TF, Stence NV, Maloney JA, et al. Pediatric brain: repeated exposure to linear gadolinium-based contrast material is associated with increased signal intensity at unenhanced T1-weighted MR imaging. Radiology 2016;160356.

41. Lanier MH, Shetty AS, Salter A, et al. Evaluation of noncontrast MR enterography for pediatric inflammatory bowel disease assessment. J Magn Reson Imaging 2018;48(2):341–8.

42. Quaia E, Sozzi M, Gennari AG, et al. Impact of gadolinium-based contrast agent in the assessment of Crohn's disease activity: is contrast agent injection necessary? J Magn Reson Imaging 2016;43(3):688–97.

43. Steward MJ, Punwani S, Proctor I, et al. Non-perforating small bowel Crohn's disease assessed by MRI enterography: derivation and histopathological validation of an MR-based activity index. Eur J Radiol 2012;81(9):2080–8.

44. Ordas I, Rimola J, Alfaro I, et al. Development and validation of a simplified magnetic resonance index of activity for Crohn's disease. Gastroenterology 2019;157(2):432–9.e1.

45. Oto A, Zhu F, Kulkarni K, et al. Evaluation of diffusion-weighted MR imaging for detection of bowel inflammation in patients with Crohn's disease. Acad Radiol 2009;16(5):597–603.

46. Oussalah A, Laurent V, Bruot O, et al. Diffusion-weighted magnetic resonance without bowel preparation for detecting colonic inflammation in inflammatory bowel disease. Gut 2010;59(8):1056–65.

47. Buisson A, Joubert A, Montoriol PF, et al. Diffusion-weighted magnetic resonance imaging for detecting and assessing ileal inflammation in Crohn's disease. Aliment Pharmacol Ther 2013;37(5):537–45.

48. Caruso A, D'Incà R, Scarpa M, et al. Diffusion-weighted magnetic resonance for assessing ileal Crohn's disease activity. Inflamm Bowel Dis 2014;20(9):1575–83.

49. Tielbeek JA, Ziech ML, Li Z, et al. Evaluation of conventional, dynamic contrast enhanced and diffusion weighted MRI for quantitative Crohn's disease assessment with histopathology of surgical specimens. Eur Radiol 2014;24(3):619–29.

50. Buisson A, Hordonneau C, Goutte M, et al. Diffusion-weighted magnetic resonance imaging is effective to detect ileocolonic ulcerations in Crohn's disease. Aliment Pharmacol Ther 2015;42(4):452–60.

51. Seo N, Park SH, Kim KJ, et al. MR enterography for the evaluation of small-bowel inflammation in Crohn disease by using diffusion-weighted imaging without intravenous contrast material: a prospective noninferiority study. Radiology 2016;278(3):762–72.

52. Kim KJ, Lee Y, Park SH, et al. Diffusion-weighted MR enterography for evaluating Crohn's disease: how does it add diagnostically to conventional MR enterography? Inflamm Bowel Dis 2015;21(1):101–9.

53. Shenoy-Bhangle AS, Nimkin K, Aranson T, et al. Value of diffusion-weighted imaging when added to magnetic resonance enterographic evaluation of Crohn disease in children. Pediatr Radiol 2016;46(1):34–42.

54. Lang RA, Buhmann S, Hopman A, et al. Cine-MRI detection of intraabdominal adhesions: correlation with intraoperative findings in 89 consecutive cases. Surg Endosc 2008;22(11):2455–61.

55. Buhmann-Kirchhoff S, Lang R, Kirchhoff C, et al. Functional cine MR imaging for the detection and mapping of intraabdominal adhesions: method and surgical correlation. Eur Radiol 2008;18(6):1215–23.

56. Torkzad MR, Vargas R, Tanaka C, et al. Value of cine MRI for better visualization of the proximal small bowel in normal individuals. Eur Radiol 2007;17(11):2964–8.

57. Menys A, Atkinson D, Odille F, et al. Quantified terminal ileal motility during MR enterography as a potential biomarker of Crohn's disease activity: a preliminary study. Eur Radiol 2012;22(11):2494–501.

58. Froehlich JM, Waldherr C, Stoupis C, et al. MR motility imaging in Crohn's disease improves lesion detection compared with standard MR imaging. Eur Radiol 2010;20(8):1945–51.

59. Hahnemann ML, Nensa F, Kinner S, et al. Improved detection of inflammatory bowel disease by additional automated motility analysis in magnetic resonance imaging. Invest Radiol 2015;50(2):67–72.

60. Bickelhaupt S, Froehlich JM, Cattin R, et al. Differentiation between active and chronic Crohn's disease using MRI smallbowel motility examinations - initial experience. Clin Radiol 2013;68(12):1247–53.

61. Cullmann JL, Bickelhaupt S, Froehlich JM, et al. MR imaging in Crohn's disease: correlation of MR motility measurement with histopathology in the terminal ileum. Neurogastroenterol Motil 2013;25(9). 749-e577.

62. Bickelhaupt S, Pazahr S, Chuck N, et al. Crohn's disease: small bowel motility impairment correlates with inflammatory-related markers C-reactive protein and calprotectin. Neurogastroenterol Motil 2013;25(6): 467–73.

63. Plumb AA, Menys A, Russo E, et al. Magnetic resonance imaging-quantified small bowel motility is a sensitive marker of response to medical therapy in Crohn's disease. Aliment Pharmacol Ther 2015; 42(3):343–55.

64. Pazahr S, Blume I, Frei P, et al. Magnetization transfer for the assessment of bowel fibrosis in patients with Crohn's disease: initial experience. MAGMA 2013;26(3):291–301.

65. Huang SY, Li XH, Huang L, et al. T2* Mapping to characterize intestinal fibrosis in crohn's disease. J Magn Reson Imaging 2018. [Epub ahead of print].

66. Sohn B, Kim MJ, Koh H, et al. Intestinal lesions in pediatric Crohn disease: comparative detectability among pulse sequences at MR enterography. Pediatr Radiol 2014;44(7):821–30.

67. Barber JL, Lozinsky AC, Kiparissi F, et al. Detecting inflammation in the unprepared pediatric colon - how reliable is magnetic resonance enterography? Pediatr Radiol 2016;46(5):646–52.

68. Absah I, Bruining DH, Matsumoto JM, et al. MR enterography in pediatric inflammatory bowel disease: retrospective assessment of patient tolerance, image quality, and initial performance estimates. AJR Am J Roentgenol 2012;199(3):W367–75.

69. Maccioni F, Al Ansari N, Mazzamurro F, et al. Detection of Crohn disease lesions of the small and large bowel in pediatric patients: diagnostic value of MR enterography versus reference examinations. AJR Am J Roentgenol 2014;203(5):W533–42.

70. Friedrich C, Fajfar A, Pawlik M, et al. Magnetic resonance enterography with and without biphasic contrast agent enema compared to conventional ileocolonoscopy in patients with Crohn's disease. Inflamm Bowel Dis 2012;18(10):1842–8.

71. Narin B, Ajaj W, Göhde S, et al. Combined small and large bowel MR imaging in patients with Crohn's disease: a feasibility study. Eur Radiol 2004;14(9): 1535–42.

72. Rimola J, Rodriguez S, García-Bosch O, et al. Magnetic resonance for assessment of disease activity and severity in ileocolonic Crohn's disease. Gut 2009;58(8):1113–20.

73. Puylaert CAJ, Schuffler PJ, Naziroglu RE, et al. Semiautomatic assessment of the terminal ileum and colon in patients with Crohn disease using MRI (the VIGOR++ Project). Acad Radiol 2018; 25(8):1038–45.

74. Taylor SA, Mallett S, Bhatnagar G, et al. Diagnostic accuracy of magnetic resonance enterography and small bowel ultrasound for the extent and activity of newly diagnosed and relapsed Crohn's disease (METRIC): a multicentre trial. Lancet Gastroenterol Hepatol 2018;3(8):548–58.

Magnetic Resonance in Crohn's Disease
Diagnosis, Disease Burden, and Classification

Luís S. Guimarães, MD, PhD[a,b], Mary-Louise C. Greer, MBBS[b,c], Jonathan R. Dillman, MD[d], Joel G. Fletcher, MD[e,*]

KEYWORDS

- Crohn's disease • MR enterography • Inflammation • Stricture • Fistula

KEY POINTS

- Magnetic resonance enterography (MRE) should be performed at the time of Crohn's diagnosis to detect small bowel inflammation, strictures, and penetrating complications that are not detected by ileocolonoscopy and serum or fecal markers.
- Active inflammatory small bowel Crohn's disease should be diagnosed when bowel wall thickening and segmental hyperenhancement coexist in a known patient with Crohn's, are present with typical penetrating or stricturing complications, or are present asymmetrically in the bowel wall along the mesenteric border.
- When small bowel Crohn's disease is present, radiologists should describe its location, length, and severity, because these important parameters influence treatment decisions.
- In the presence of a stricture (defined as an area of diseased luminal narrowing associated with un-equivocal upstream dilatation >3 cm), presence of active inflammation, length, degree of upstream dilatation, presence of associated penetrating complications, and enteric anastomoses should be described.
- Expected areas of advancement including MRE involve development of (1) biomarkers capable of predicting drug response and outcomes, (2) pulse sequences able to measure wall fibrosis, (3) classifiers of disease using MRE pulse sequences without the use of intravenous contrast.

INTRODUCTION

Crohn's disease (CD) is a chronic inflammatory condition involving predominantly the gastrointestinal (GI) tract, with increasing incidence worldwide. Recently developed targeted biologic agents result in the ability to improve long-term outcomes and reduce patient morbidity.

Consequently, there is a growing need to monitor drug and antibody levels and predict (and ensure) treatment response. Deep and long-lasting remission from enteric inflammation is the goal of therapy, and therapeutic monitoring can avoid underuse and detect nonresponse. Besides imaging, the main tools gastroenterologists have at

Disclosure: The authors have nothing to disclose.
[a] Joint Department of Medical Imaging, Sinai Health System, UHN and Women's College Hospital, Toronto, ON, Canada; [b] Department of Medical Imaging, University of Toronto, 4th Floor, 263 McCaul Street, Toronto, ON M5T 1W7, Canada; [c] Department of Diagnostic Imaging, The Hospital for Sick Children, 555 University Avenue, Toronto, ON M5G 1X8, Canada; [d] Department of Radiology, Cincinnati Children's Hospital, 3333 Burnet Avenue, Cincinnati, OH 45229, USA; [e] Department of Radiology, Mayo Clinic, 200 First Street Southwest, Rochester, MN 55905, USA
* Corresponding author.
E-mail address: fletcher.joel@mayo.edu

Magn Reson Imaging Clin N Am 28 (2020) 31–44
https://doi.org/10.1016/j.mric.2019.08.003
1064-9689/20/© 2019 Elsevier Inc. All rights reserved.

hand are patient symptoms, therapeutic drug monitoring, endoscopic/histologic assessment, and serum/fecal markers. However, many symptomatic indices are prone to interobserver variability, incorporate subjective terms such as well-being or abdominal pain, and do not reflect objective markers of inflammation burden such as endoscopy and histology. Consequently, additional objective measures of active disease, response to treatment, and complications are needed.

Magnetic resonance enterography (MRE) is now an established test in patients with Crohn's because of its ability to show transmural enteric inflammation and treatment response throughout the GI tract without the very low potential risk of ionizing radiation. This article provides a road map for how and when to diagnose CD with MRE (including discussion of the main differential diagnoses), how to describe the burden of enteric inflammation and its complications, and how to accurately classify disease based on interdisciplinary consensus. In addition, brief overviews of expected future MRE developments and alternative imaging modalities are also discussed.

ADAPTATION TO STANDARD IMAGING PROTOCOLS

Optimal small bowel magnetic resonance (MR) imaging protocols in general are discussed comprehensively elsewhere (see Darren Boone and Stuart A. Taylor's article, "MR of the Small Bowel: How to Do It," in this issue). Recommendations on MRE protocols have been published by the Society of Abdominal Radiology (SAR)[1] and by the European Society of Gastrointestinal and Abdominal Radiology (ESGAR) in consensus with the European Crohn's and Colitis Organisation (ECCO) (**Table 1**).[2] Specific considerations based on patient age and on particular clinical questions (presence of perianal disease or existence of significant fibrosis in Crohn's lesions) are discussed later.

Adaptations for the pediatric population

Patient cooperation is essential to achieving diagnostic quality MRE in children and adolescents.[3] Education preceding MRE, and active encouragement during the examination, can optimize compliance by helping ensure proper fasting for 4 to 6 hours, drinking the required volume of enteric contrast material, staying still, and good breath holding.[4]

Weight-based protocols are used in pediatric patients to determine the volumes of enteric and intravenous (IV) gadolinium-based contrast agents (GBCAs) and dose of antispasmodic agent

administered. Enteric contrast is administered as 3 boluses over 45 to 60 minutes.[5] Providing patients with a choice of enteric contrast agents improves compliance.[6,7] These hyperosmolar contrast agents provide comparable but improved distension compared with water and are often more palatable when chilled.[4,6,7]

The antispasmodic agents glucagon and hyoscine-butyl-bromide (Buscopan) are both used in pediatric patients; Buscopan is off label in children but may be slightly better tolerated.[4] These agents are administered as 1 or 2 doses before GBCA.[4]

Imaging acquisition following intravenous GBCA injections can be dynamic postcontrast, enteric phase (45 seconds), portal venous phase (70 seconds), and/or delayed up to 7 minutes, similar to adults.[5,8]

Imaging sequences used in pediatric MRE are the same as those detailed for adult MRE protocols, with acquisition parameters adapted to patient size. General anesthesia may be needed for MRE in younger patients (eg, <6 years old) and in those with impaired cognition or developmental delay.[9] Modifications for general anesthesia include intubation; enteric contrast given via orogastric or transpyloric tube in multiple doses before image acquisition; and avoidance of antispasmodic agents, which can potentiate anesthesia-related ileus.[10,11]

Combined magnetic resonance enterography and perianal protocols

Standard MRE protocols are useful to screen the perianal region (the perianal region should be imaged as part of standard MRE examinations), but may not completely exclude or classify perianal fistulas without dedicated pelvic/perianal imaging.[12,13] AlSabban and colleagues[12] found that MRE had a high sensitivity of 82% and very high specificity of 100% for detection of any perianal disease, but did not identify some fistulae and small-volume abscesses, so MRE also is insufficient for fistula classification (**Fig. 1**).[14] There is an additional time penalty by combining pelvic MR imaging with MRE that can result in increased motion artifacts or be complicated by incontinence; however, adding a limited number of small-field-of-view, multiplanar T2-weighted images to routine MRE may improve fistula detection.[15]

Techniques for identification of bowel wall fibrosis

The presence of strictures is commonly an indication for endoscopic or surgical intervention, and

Table 1
Protocol suggestions by Society of Abdominal Radiology and European Crohn's and Colitis Organisation–European Society of Gastrointestinal and Abdominal Radiology consensus

	SAR	ECCO-ESGAR[2]
Patient preparation	• Fasting for 2–4 h	• Fasting for 4–6 h
Equipment	• Not mentioned	• ≥1.5 T magnet • Phased array coils
Anatomic coverage	• Include entire small/large bowel + anal region,[a] even if excluding part of liver/spleen	• Not mentioned

Bowel paralysis	• Recommended
	  ○ Glucagon or butylscopolamine
		• Recommended
		  ○ Butylscopolamine agent of choice, glucagon an alternative

Enteric contrast	• Biphasic iso-osmotic/hyperosmotic enteric contrast (eg, Volumen, Breeza, PEG, methylcellulose) • >900 mL (as much as possible up to 2 L) • 45–60 min before scanning • Rectal contrast provides better colonic assessment, but not routine	• Hyperosmotic enteric contrast (eg, sorbitol solution, PEG) • >1000 mL if possible, any better than nothing • 45 min before scanning • Rectal contrast provides better colonic assessment, but not routine
Mandatory sequences	• T2-weighted axial and coronal, 1 plane with fat saturation • Dynamic contrast-enhanced coronal T1-weighted fat-saturated 3D GRE: acquire at 45 s with 2 subsequent coronal acquisitions • Axial contrast-enhanced T1-weighted fat-saturated 3D GRE	• T2-weighted and BSSFP • Dynamic contrast-enhanced coronal T1 weighted at enteric or portal venous phase should be always considered, but use decided on a patient-by-patient basis • DWI/cine BSSFP if intravenous contrast not used
Optional sequences	• BSSFP (highly recommended, excellent for anatomy depiction) • DWI • Magnetization transfer • Delayed contrast enhanced (at 5–7 min) • Cine BSSFP	• DWI • Cine BSSFP

Abbreviations: 3D, three-dimensional; BSSFP, balanced steady state free precession; DWI, diffusion-weighted imaging; GRE, gradient echo; PEG, polyethylene glycol.

[a] Routine MRE protocols do not thoroughly delineate perianal fistulae and their relationship to the sphincteric complexes, but can detect/exclude most penetrating complications.

Adapted from Grand DJ, Guglielmo FF, Al-Hawary MM. MR enterography in Crohn's disease: current consensus on optimal imaging technique and future advances from the SAR Crohn's disease-focused panel. Abdom Imaging 2015;40(5):954; with permission.

the ability to detect and measure intestinal fibrosis in strictures would be helpful for directing the medical and surgical management; however, fibrosis is challenging to identify using conventional MR imaging techniques.

Barkmeier and colleagues[16] concluded that the degree of small bowel dilatation proximal to an area of luminal narrowing of more than 3 cm was highly associated with confluent transmural fibrosis on histopathologic assessment following stricture resection (**Fig. 2**). Rimola and colleagues[8] evaluated change in bowel wall enhancement over time and found that progressive stricture enhancement between 70 seconds and 7 minutes and homogeneous enhancement on delayed images correlate with histologic fibrosis. Animal as well as human studies have also suggested that magnetization transfer (MT) MR imaging can be used to detect and estimate the amount of bowel wall fibrosis. Increased macromolecule concentration, such as collagen, causes a tissue's MT ratio (MTR) to increase, allowing MTR to be used as a surrogate for bowel wall fibrosis. Li and colleagues have extended prior work and shown that MTRs

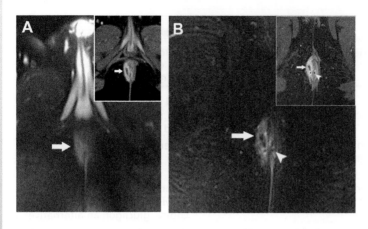

Fig. 1. – MRE image (*A*) shows right perianal fistula (*arrow*), but subsequent dedicated pelvic MR imaging (*B*) better shows fistula morphology (*arrow*) and seton (*arrowhead*).

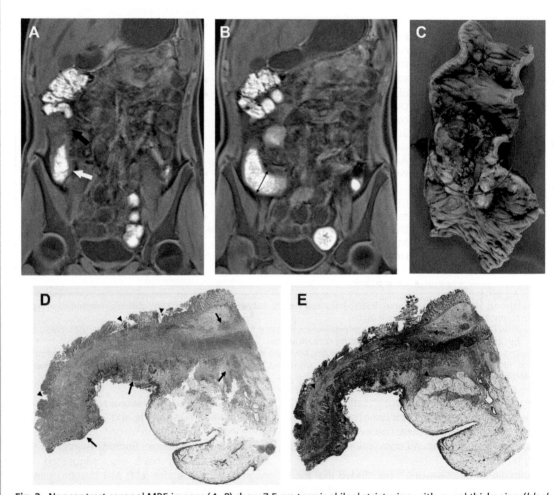

Fig. 2. Noncontrast coronal MRE images (*A, B*) show 7.5-cm terminal ileal stricturing with mural thickening (*black arrow*) and upstream fecalization (*white arrow*), with 3.8-cm prestenotic dilatation (*double-headed arrow*). (*C*) Surgical ileocecectomy specimen shows the stricture (*circle*). (*D*) Histopathology images using hematoxylin-eosin staining show ulceration (*arrowheads*) and submucosal and deep subserosal lymphoid aggregates (*arrows*). (*E*) Masson elastic trichrome stain shows mural expansion with bands of submucosal and subserosal collagen (*arrowheads*). (D&E, original magnification ×2). ([*C–E*] *Courtesy of* I. Siddiqui, MBBS, MSc, FRCPC, Toronto, Canada.)

normalized to skeletal muscle are significantly higher in fibrotic bowel segments in patients with CD.[17-19] Ultimately, additional research is needed to establish which of these methods is best for detecting and measuring bowel wall fibrosis.

IMAGING FINDINGS AND PATHOLOGY
Crohn's Disease and How It Affects the Bowel

CD is one of the major subtypes of inflammatory bowel disease (IBD) and is characterized by active, chronic, relapsing inflammation of the GI tract, of multifactorial cause including different genotypes, with several monogenetic mutations now recognized in children less than 6 years old with very-early-onset IBD (VEO-IBD).[3,20-22] Although ulcerative colitis (UC) is limited to the colon, CD can affect anywhere from the mouth to the anus, most often small and large bowel (usually discontinuous), involves the adjacent mesentery, with inflammation often more pronounced along the mesenteric border. At a microscopic level, active inflammation of the GI tract in CD is seen as a patchy transmural process, with the presence of nonnecrotizing, noncryptolytic epithelioid granulomas in mucosal and/or submucosal lymphoid tissue, pivotal to distinguishing CD from UC.[23]

Bowel wall inflammation variably progresses to stricturing and/or penetrating disease, the hallmarks of CD (typically a transmural process), differing in number of involved segments, location, extent, and severity over time and between patients.

The Montreal and Paris classification systems are used to define the spectrum of different CD phenotypes seen in adults and children, respectively,[24,25] but do not adequately summarize the coexistence of inflammation, inflammation severity, and stricturing/penetrating complications seen on MRE.

Crohn's Disease Presentation, Progression and Stricture Formation

Classic clinical findings of CD are abdominal pain, diarrhea, and weight loss, but few patients have all three at presentation, often leading to a delay in diagnosis.[3] Unexplained anemia presenting as fatigue, fever, and linear growth impairment warrant particular attention in children, as does secondary amenorrhea.[3] Around 20% to 26% of adults initially present with a penetrating or obstructing complication compared with approximately 10% in children, who may also present with cutaneous CD.[26,27] Disease progression varies with time, therapy, and location, with ileal disease more often leading to stricture (from smooth muscle hypertrophy and collagen deposition) and pseudosacculation.[21,24] Obstruction, with worsening pain and

vomiting, can occur with bowel wall thickening and edema from active bowel inflammation or mixed inflammatory and fibrotic strictures (see **Fig. 2**).

Spectrum of Penetrating Disease

Penetrating disease occurs with progression of CD, more often in patients having frequent flares, and manifests as sinus tracts, fistulas, inflammatory masses, and abscesses, being accurately detected with contrast-enhanced MRE (**Fig. 3**).[13,21,28] Recent data have shown that internal penetrating disease is associated with luminal narrowing/bowel stricturing and sites of active bowel inflammation.[29]

Associations with Perianal Disease

VEO-IBD is very rare (3%) but colonic and especially perianal disease predominates in this setting.[20,22] Although perianal disease is present in a substantial minority of children and adults at diagnosis, it may be the only manifestation of CD in 5%.[3] The incidence of perianal disease increases the closer colonic inflammation is located to the anus, and perianal fistulas do not heal when proctitis is present. In children, a distinct phenotype is characterized by perianal disease in conjunction with an overall worse burden of rectal and jejunal inflammation.[30]

Other Perienteric/Extraintestinal Complications

Perienteric features of CD can be a sign or a sequela of active inflammation, and include regional fibrofatty proliferation, also known as creeping fat; engorgement of the vasa recta, or "comb" sign; mesenteric enhancement and edema; and, rarely, mesenteric venous thrombosis if acute, and mesenteric venous occlusions with or without varices if chronic.[13] Extraintestinal manifestations of CD include gallstones, renal stones, pancreatitis (eg, autoimmune or caused by immunosuppression with azathioprine) and spondyloarthritis, and can be detected with MRE. Primary sclerosing cholangitis occurs most commonly in conjunction with IBD, and is of prognostic importance because of poor survival outcomes; therefore suspicion of intrahepatic or extrahepatic bile duct dilatation or beading on MRE should prompt dedicated imaging with magnetic resonance cholangiopancreatography.[13]

DIAGNOSTIC CRITERIA

MR imaging features correlating best with active inflammatory CD of the bowel include segmental

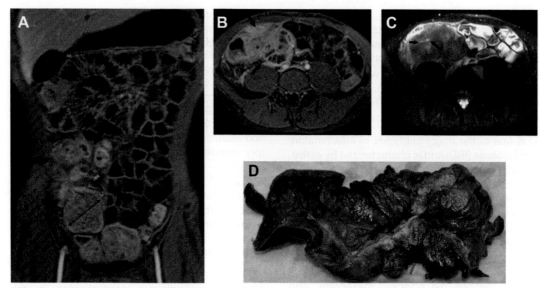

Fig. 3. (*A-C*) MRE images show a complex inflammatory mass in the right lower quadrant (*black arrows* in *A* and *B*) medial to the thick-walled ileocecal region with terminal ileal narrowing and prestenotic ileal dilatation (*A*) measuring 5.5 cm (*double-headed arrow*), with suspicion of sinus tracts in the wall (*arrows* in *C*), but no drainable abscess. (*D*) Surgical ileocecectomy specimen shows 8-cm stricture with perforation and a healed fissuring ulcer (*arrow*). ([*D*] *Courtesy of* I. Siddiqui, MBBS, MSc, FRCPC, Toronto, Canada.)

mural hyperenhancement and mural thickening, especially if asymmetric (affecting predominantly the mesenteric border), T2-weighted signal hyperintensity (reflecting intramural edema),[31] restricted diffusion on diffusion-weighted imaging (DWI), and luminal ulcers (breaks in the inner wall of the small bowel with associated intramural extension of air or enteric contrast (**Figs. 4** and **5**).[13,32] These imaging findings correlate with endoscopic and histologic evidence of active inflammation in adults and children, and are reflected in MR imaging indices used to score inflammatory disease severity such as the MR index of activity and London scores.[28,33–35] Because imaging findings are

frequently nonspecific,[36] intersociety recommendations state that active inflammatory Crohn's small bowel disease should be diagnosed when bowel wall thickening and segmental hyperenhancement coexist in a known patient with Crohn's, are present with typical penetrating or stricturing complications, or are present asymmetrically in the bowel wall predominantly along the mesenteric border (see **Figs. 5** and **6**, **Table 2**).[13] Restricted diffusion is not part of the diagnostic criteria for CD but reflects inflammation severity (see **Fig. 4**).[13,37,38] In the jejunum, asymmetric inflammation distorts or effaces the normal fold pattern (see **Figs. 6** and **7**). Nonspecific imaging findings

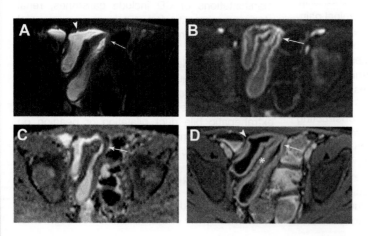

Fig. 4. (*A–D*) MRE images in a pediatric patient show severe active bowel wall inflammation shown by (*A*) intramural T2-weighted signal hyperintensity (*arrow*), (*B, C*) restricted diffusion (*arrows*), (*D*) hyperenhancement (*arrow*) with bowel wall thickening (*asterisk*) and (*A* and *D*) luminal ulceration (*arrowheads*).

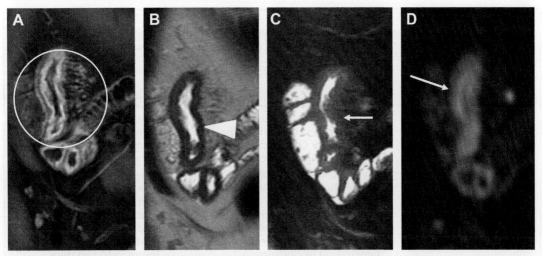

Fig. 5. (*A–D*) MRE images in an adult patient show segmental mural hyperenhancement and wall thickening in the terminal ileum with (*A*) engorged vasa recta (*circle*), (*B*) wall thickening with luminal ulceration (*arrowhead*), and (*C, D*) marked increase in intramural T2 hyperintensity and restricted diffusion (*arrows*).

can be correlated with clinical symptoms and endoscopic findings and followed over time to determine their import.

Identification of Crohn's strictures is important because stricture formation leads to obstructing complications, and most penetrating complications are associated with luminal narrowing or overt strictures.[29] Although MRE is highly accurate in identifying Crohn's strictures, consistent use of specific imaging criteria has been lacking.[39] Society of Abdominal Radiology (SAR) and American Gastroenterological Association (AGA) consensus recommendations have defined a small bowel stricture as an area of luminal narrowing in a bowel segment affected by CD associated with unequivocal upstream dilatation greater than 3 cm (**Figs. 8 and 9**).[13,29] An expert consensus panel recently refined this definition to include a 50% decrease in luminal diameter inside the stricture, a 25% increase in wall thickness, and proximal small bowel dilatation of at least 3 cm.[40] A probable stricture is present when luminal narrowing and wall

thickening are combined with unequivocal proximal small bowel dilatation on multiple studies or multiple pulse sequences. In applying MRE definitions, it should be remembered that luminal obstruction is a dynamic process, and that the proximal small bowel dilatation varies over the course of an examination as the enteric bolus travels through the small bowel, so the greatest measurement should be used.

DIFFERENTIAL DIAGNOSIS

At initial/acute presentation, imaging findings may be nonspecific and the list of diseases causing similar findings can be broad, including infectious processes and bowel ischemia; in these situations, clinical features are usually more revealing than imaging findings. Similarly, entities that primarily occur in immunocompromised patients are rarely assessed with MR imaging. However, there are several diseases that may present with at least some of the imaging features that are

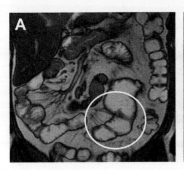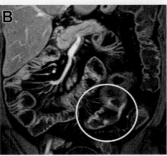

Fig. 6. (*A*) Coronal TrueFISP (true fast imaging with steady state precession) and (*B*) postgadolinium images show mild but diagnostic CD manifested by effacement of jejunal folds and patchy, asymmetric wall thickening, and enhancement (*circles*).

Table 2
Diagnostic criteria for active inflammatory small bowel Crohn's disease manifestations at magnetic resonance enterography and required elements (necessary modifiers) that assist with therapeutic decision making

Imaging Conclusion/ Descriptor	Diagnostic Criteria	Necessary Modifiers
Nonspecific inflammation	• Symmetric mural hyperenhancement and wall thickening without prior Crohn's diagnosis or penetrating complications	• Location • Length • Patency of mesenteric vessels, presence of ascites

Active inflammatory small bowel CD	• Asymmetric/patchy mural hyperenhancement and wall thickening
	• Symmetric hyperenhancement and wall thickening with prior diagnosis of Crohn's or typical penetrating or obstructing complications
		• Location
		• Length
		• Severity
		  Mild: 3–5 mm thick
		  Moderate: 5–10 mm thick, intramural edema
		  Severe: ≥10 mm thick, luminal ulcerations, diffusion restriction, intramural edema

Stricture	• Luminal narrowing + wall thickening + unequivocal proximal small bowel dilatation of ≥3 cm, or inability to pass endoscope combined with luminal narrowing, wall thickening, proximal small bowel dilatation (<3 cm) • Probable strictures noted if proximal small bowel dilatation of 2.5–3.0 cm, or stricture shown on prior CTE/MRE	• State whether imaging findings of inflammation are present or not • Associated with enteric anastomosis • Length • Maximal degree (in cm) of proximal small bowel dilatation shown in any plane • Associated penetrating complications
Penetrating complications	• Sinus tract • Simple fistula • Complex fistula • Inflammatory mass • Abscess	• State whether abscess is present or absent • State whether a fistula is simple or complex • Describe association with stricture/inflamed segment, or anastomosis • Describe all ramifications and extensions • If associated with stricture, describe proximal small bowel dilatation

Abbreviation: CTE, computed tomography enterography.
Adapted from Bruining DH, Zimmermann EM, Loftus EV, et al. Consensus Recommendations for Evaluation, Interpretation, and Utilization of Computed Tomography and Magnetic Resonance Enterography in Patients With Small Bowel Crohn's Disease. Radiology 2018;286(3):793; with permission.

typically considered to be relatively specific of CD, such as multiple skip lesions showing mural thickening and hyperenhancement, sometimes associated with luminal stenosis or strictures (Fig. 10). Distinction between CD and these entities is typically based on a combination of clinical and imaging features. Table 3 summarizes important differences, both clinical and MRE features, that can aid in distinguishing between CD and entities that may present with multiple (skip) bowel lesions showing mural thickening/hyperenhancement and luminal stenosis/strictures.

DESCRIBING CROHN'S DISEASE BURDEN AND CLASSIFICATION

When small bowel CD is present, radiologists should describe its location, length, and severity,

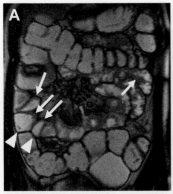
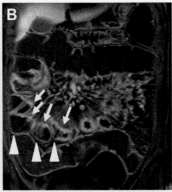

Fig. 7. (*A*) Coronal TrueFISP and (*B*) postgadolinium images show extensive jejunal disease manifested by patchy diffuse wall thickening, distortion of jejunal folds, and segmental hyperenhancement with engorged vasa recta. Note the asymmetry of the process, with the mesenteric border (*arrows*) significantly more involved than the antimesenteric border (*arrowheads*).

because these important parameters influence treatment decisions. For instance, duodenal Crohn's is often associated with stricture formation and obstruction,[41] whereas jejunal involvement is a marker for extensive small bowel involvement and increases the risk of surgery and hospitalization.[42] As another example, the length of small bowel inflammation is a critical and underemphasized feature of Crohn's, but directly communicates the amount of gut that is at risk for progressive destruction and is a marker for response to treatment or worsening.[43] Based on these findings, specific impression statements can be generated and added to the imaging report (see **Table 2**).[13] An increase in the number and severity of findings of intestinal and mesenteric inflammation subjectively suggests worsening intestinal active inflammation.

In a considerable number of patients with CD, ongoing intestinal inflammation leads to stricture formation. The presence of active inflammation associated with the strictured bowel segment should always be described, because antiinflammatory therapies may decrease the obstructive component and penetrating complications often arise from strictures with inflammation (see **Fig 8**).[29] Additional key features of CD strictures to evaluate include length of the narrowed bowel segment, degree of upstream dilatation, and presence of associated penetrating complications or enteric anastomoses (see **Table 2**).[13] Length is a key feature because short strictures may be amenable to balloon dilatation (if <5 cm) or bowel-preserving strictureplasty. Anastomotic strictures may represent a unique subtype of CD stricture arising from local intestinal ischemia and/or CD inflammation. A systematic description of other imaging features of CD strictures is currently lacking, but when there is a small number of strictures (eg, 2 or 3) each should be described separately. In patients with numerous strictures (eg, 6–

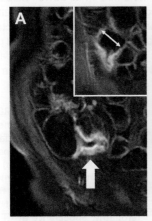
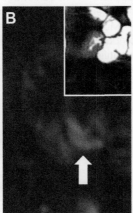
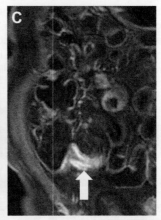

Fig. 8. (*A*) Coronal MRE images show a neoterminal ileal stricture at the ileocecal anastomosis (*arrow*) with marked luminal narrowing, wall thickening, and proximal small bowel dilatation to 3.2 cm (*inset, double headed arrow*). (*B*) Increased DWI signal abnormality and intramural edema indicate inflammation within the stricture, and (*C*) delayed gadolinium image shows progressive but layered enhancement, likely indicating both inflammation and fibrosis are present (*arrows*).

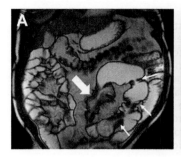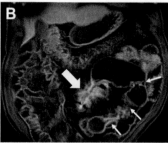

Fig. 9. (*A, B*) MRE images show multifocal small bowel strictures (*thin arrows*) of different lengths with the dominant stricture (*thick arrows*) showing the greatest degree of proximal small bowel dilatation.

10), the approximate number of strictures should be described as well as the bowel segments involved (eg, proximal jejunum, midileum; see **Fig. 9**). In patients with numerous strictures, the most dominant strictures (with greatest proximal small bowel dilatation) should be described in detail at a minimum.

Penetrating disease most often arises from the proximal or midportion of an inflamed, narrowed bowel segment.[29] Each identified penetrating complication (blind-ending sinus tracts, fistulas, inflammatory masses, and abscesses) should be described, including the portions of the bowel involved as well as involvement of extraenteric structures (eg, abdominal wall, urinary bladder). More than 1 penetrating complication is present in some patients, with complex, stellate-shaped fistulas often giving rise to multiple fistulous tracts (the star sign) with a central interloop abscess (**Fig. 11**).

USE

Without correlative cross-sectional imaging at the time of diagnosis, it is estimated that approximately one-third of patients have undetected penetrating or obstructing complications.[44] Moreover, in patients with known Crohn's, computed tomography enterography (CTE) or MRE identifies small bowel inflammation not seen at ileoscopy

about 50% of the time,[45–47] primarily because of intramural inflammation (with overlying normal mucosa), proximal small bowel inflammation, stenosis at the ileocecal valve or anastomosis, or penetrating complications.

For these reasons, intersociety consensus statements recommend MRE for patients with suspected Crohn's at time of diagnosis, and for assessment of therapeutic response in patients with small bowel CD.[13] In this context, serum tests and fecal markers are also used to follow patients, with MRE often being used to assess inflammation when drug levels are appropriate and antidrug antibody levels are low.[48] Cross-sectional enterography changes management decisions in about half of patients with Crohn's even when ileoscopic results are known,[49] and therapeutic response as assessed by CTE/MRE has been shown to predict patient outcomes.[50–52]

ALTERNATIVE IMAGING STRATEGIES

MRE is often preferred to bowel ultrasonography or CTE in patients with small bowel CD because it can image the entire small bowel, displays multiple imaging findings reflecting inflammation severity (ulcers, intramural edema, restricted diffusion), does not use ionizing radiation, and provides an excellent method to screen for perianal disease.[13] Low-radiation-dose CTE is medically

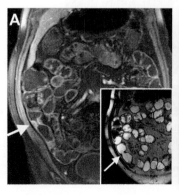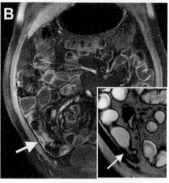

Fig. 10. (*A, B*) Coronal MRE images show 2 nearby short-segment strictures typical of nonsteroidal antiinflammatory drug enteropathy on coronal postcontrast (*arrows*) and precontrast TrueFISP images (*inset, small arrows*). (Adapted from Frye JM, Hansel SL, Dolan SG, et al. NSAID enteropathy: appearance at CT and MR enterography in the age of multimodality imaging and treatment. Abdom Imaging 2015;40(5):1020; with permission.)

Table 3
Clinical and imaging features useful for the distinction between Crohn's disease and other entities that may present with multiple (skip) bowel lesions showing mural thickening/hyperenhancement and luminal stenosis/strictures

	Differentiating Clinical Features	Differentiating Imaging Features
NSAID enteropathy	• Frequently >50 y old • Chronic intake of NSAIDs (disclosed or not) • Prior negative work-up including upper and lower endoscopy • Absence of perianal disease	• Diaphragmlike or ringlike circumferential very short (5–10 mm) lesions • Symmetric with respect to the bowel lumen • Absence of colonic involvement, terminal ileum rarely involved

CMUSE	• Prior negative work-up including upper and lower endoscopy
	• Absence of clinical or laboratory features of an inflammatory condition
	• No extraintestinal manifestations
	• Absence of perianal disease
		• Short and thin strictures (mean length ≈1 cm)
		• Features atypical of CMUSE:
		  ○ Significant bowel obstruction
		  ○ Penetrating disease
		  ○ Mesenteric stranding
		  ○ Lymphadenopathy
		• No GI involvement besides small bowel

Tuberculosis	• Diarrhea, hematochezia, presence of perianal disease, and extraintestinal manifestations are rare
	• High fever, night sweats, lung involvement, and ascites more common
	• Duration of symptoms usually shorter than in Crohn's disease
	• Absence of perianal disease
		• Necrotic lymph nodes are distinctive feature
		• Peritoneal thickening (even omental caking) may be seen
		• Following features are rare in tuberculosis:
		  ○ Skip lesions
		  ○ Asymmetric strictures with pseudosacculation along antimesenteric border
		  ○ Fibrofatty proliferation
		  ○ Penetrating disease
		  ○ Left colon involvement

Behçet disease	• Typically recurrent oral ulcerations plus 2 of the following: recurrent genital ulcerations, eye lesions, skin lesions, positive results from a pathergy test, neurologic and vascular involvement • Absence of perianal disease (<1%)	• Polypoid masslike changes more common than in CD • Perforation common • Except for complicated cases, perienteric changes usually minimal

HSP	• Virtually all patients develop palpable purpura
	  ○ Skin biopsy shows dermal vascular IgA and complement deposition with leukocytoclastic vasculitis
	• Joint and renal involvement more common
	• Resolves more quickly and less prone to relapse
	• Absence of perianal disease
		• Intussusception much more common
		• Following features are rare in HSP:
		  ○ Significant bowel obstruction (except if intussusception)
		  ○ Penetrating disease (virtually never)
		  ○ Lymphadenopathy
		  ○ GI involvement besides small bowel

Endometriosis	• Symptoms of bowel endometriosis can be associated with the patient's menstrual cycle
	• Absence of clinical or laboratory features of an inflammatory condition
	• Absence of perianal disease
		• Endometrial implants typically located on the antimesenteric border of the bowel
		• Deposits usually in the pelvis
		• Deposits with variable appearance, but usually:
		  ○ Absence of multilayered pattern of enhancement
		  ○ More masslike than CD

Abbreviations: CMUSE, cryptogenic multifocal ulcerous stenosing enteritis; HSP, Henoch-Schönlein purpura; IgA, immunoglobulin A; NSAID, nonsteroidal antiinflammatory drug.

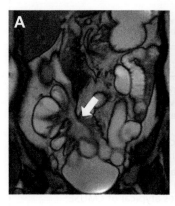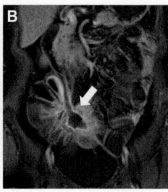

Fig. 11. (*A*) Coronal TrueFISP and (*B*) postgadolinium images show complex, stellate-shaped fistula tethering multiple small bowel loops and the bladder dome with an interloop abscess (*arrows*).

justified in symptomatic patients, available in emergent settings, and performs equivalently to MRE for identifying active inflammation, strictures, and penetrating complications. A recent multicenter study found that the sensitivity and specificity of MRE was higher than that of bowel ultrasonography even in experienced hands[53]; however, ultrasonography may be a quicker and cheaper alternative to assess for therapeutic response in some patients. In addition, in patients with mild inflammation without stricturing lesions, capsule endoscopy identifies active small bowel CD, particularly in the jejunum, which can be missed at cross-sectional imaging studies, and is a complimentary tool in such patients.

SUMMARY AND FUTURE DIRECTIONS

The role of cross-sectional enterography has significantly evolved in the last decade, and multiple interdisciplinary consensus recommendations currently state that MRE has an essential role in diagnosing and monitoring response in CD. This consensus results from multiple factors, including:

1. The poor correlation between patient symptoms and the existence of bowel inflammation/damage
2. The complementarity between endoscopy and imaging for CD diagnosis, staging, and monitoring
3. The evolution of a more effective therapeutic armamentarium
4. The benefits of deep, long-lasting control of the inflammation for patient outcomes
5. The technical evolution and availability of magnetic resonance scanners and standardization of protocols

However, there are still significant challenges in CD and a growing potential for new roles for imaging. For instance, there is an unmet need for biomarkers capable of predicting drug response and patient outcomes. Use of radiomics and deep convolutional neural networks combined with imaging and other clinical information may have a role in the future considering the potential these emerging technologies have shown in the oncologic setting. Reliable measurement of fibrotic (collagen) burden within CD strictures might improve outcomes if antifibrotic drugs prove useful in CD. MR imaging methods such as MT, advanced DWI sequences, and T1 relaxometry may provide more quantitative insights into the presence of increased bowel wall collagen and deserve further investigation. In addition, because of the increasing awareness and uncertainty related to the potential toxicity of gadolinium deposition in the human body, there is an increasing need to find classifiers of disease using MRE sequences without the use of IV contrast. In addition, MR imaging protocols are also expected to become shorter and more quantitative in the future as a value-based culture and economic/time constraints place increasing pressure on radiology departments.

In summary, MRE has an established role in CD diagnosis and monitoring, but there are exciting novel opportunities for additional impact. The authors predict MRE will have even more significant roles in the near future, continuing to add benefit and value to patients with CD.

REFERENCES

1. Grand DJ, Guglielmo FF, Al-Hawary MM. MR enterography in Crohn's disease: current consensus on optimal imaging technique and future advances from the SAR Crohn's disease-focused panel. Abdom Imaging 2015;40(5):953–64.
2. Sturm A, Maaser C, Calabrese E, et al. ECCO-ESGAR guideline for diagnostic assessment in IBD part 2: IBD scores and general principles and technical aspects. J Crohn's Colitis 2019;13(3):273–84.

3. Levine A, Koletzko S, Turner D, et al. ESPGHAN revised porto criteria for the diagnosis of inflammatory bowel disease in children and adolescents. J Pediatr Gastroenterol Nutr 2014;58(6): 795–806.

4. Greer ML. How we do it: MR enterography. Pediatr Radiol 2016;46(6):818–28.

5. Greer MC. Paediatric magnetic resonance enterography in inflammatory bowel disease. Eur J Radiol 2018;102:129–37.

6. Dillman JR, Towbin AJ, Imbus R, et al. Comparison of two neutral oral contrast agents in pediatric patients: a prospective randomized study. Radiology 2018;288(1):245–51.

7. Gottumukkala RV, LaPointe A, Sargent D, et al. Comparison of three oral contrast preparations for magnetic resonance enterography in pediatric patients with known or suspected Crohn's disease: a prospective randomized trial. Pediatr Radiol 2019; 49(7):889–96.

8. Rimola J, Planell N, Rodriguez S, et al. Characterization of inflammation and fibrosis in Crohn's disease lesions by magnetic resonance imaging. Am J Gastroenterol 2015;110(3):432–40.

9. Torkzad MR, Masselli G, Halligan S, et al. Indications and selection of MR enterography vs. MR enteroclysis with emphasis on patients who need small bowel MRI and general anaesthesia: results of a survey. Insights Imaging 2015;6(3):339–46.

10. Anupindi SA, Podbersky DJ, Towbin AJ, et al. Pediatric inflammatory bowel disease: imaging issues with targeted solutions. Abdom Imaging 2015; 40(5):975–92.

11. Mollard BJ, Smith EA, Lai ME, et al. MR enterography under the age of 10 years: a single institutional experience. Pediatr Radiol 2016;46(1):43–9.

12. AlSabban Z, Carman N, Moineddin R, et al. Can MR enterography screen for perianal disease in pediatric inflammatory bowel disease? J Magn Reson Imaging 2018;47(6):1638–45.

13. Bruining DH, Zimmermann EM, Loftus EV Jr, et al. Consensus recommendations for evaluation, interpretation, and utilization of computed tomography and magnetic resonance enterography in patients with small bowel Crohn's disease. Radiology 2018; 286(3):776–99.

14. Hammer MR, Dillman JR, Smith EA, et al. Magnetic resonance imaging of perianal and perineal crohn disease in children and adolescents. Magn Reson Imaging Clin N Am 2013;21(4):813–28.

15. Wang G, Gee MS. A combined MR enterography-perianal MRI protocol is feasible and improves perianal disease evaluation over standard MRE in pediatric Crohn's disease patients. Paper presented at: Society for Pediatric Radiology Annual Meeting & Categorical Course 2017. Vancouver, British Columbia, May 16-20, 2017.

16. Barkmeier DT, Dillman JR, Al-Hawary M, et al. MR enterography-histology comparison in resected pediatric small bowel Crohn's disease strictures: can imaging predict fibrosis? Pediatr Radiol 2016; 46(4):498–507.

17. Li XH, Mao R, Huang SY, et al. Characterization of degree of intestinal fibrosis in patients with Crohn's disease by using magnetization transfer MR imaging. Radiology 2018;287(2):494–503.

18. Adler J, Swanson SD, Schmiedlin-Ren P, et al. Magnetization transfer helps detect intestinal fibrosis in an animal model of Crohn's disease. Radiology 2011;259(1):127–35.

19. Dillman JR, Swanson SD, Johnson LA, et al. Comparison of noncontrast MRI magnetization transfer and T2 -Weighted signal intensity ratios for detection of bowel wall fibrosis in a Crohn's disease animal model. J Magn Reson Imaging 2015;42(3): 801–10.

20. Bequet E, Sarter H, Fumery M, et al. Incidence and phenotype at diagnosis of very-early-onset compared with later-onset paediatric inflammatory bowel disease: a population-based study [1988-2011]. J Crohn's Colitis 2017;11(5):519–26.

21. Louis E, Michel V, Hugot JP, et al. Early development of stricturing or penetrating pattern in Crohn's disease is influenced by disease location, number of flares, and smoking but not by NOD2/CARD15 genotype. Gut 2003;52(4):552–7.

22. Watson TA, Petit P, Augdal TA, et al. European Society of Paediatric Radiology abdominal imaging task force: statement on imaging in very early onset inflammatory bowel disease. Pediatr Radiol 2019; 49(6):841–8.

23. Feakins RM. Ulcerative colitis or Crohn's disease? Pitfalls and problems. Histopathology 2014;64(3): 317–35.

24. Hyams JS. Standardized recording of parameters related to the natural history of inflammatory bowel disease: from Montreal to Paris. Dig Dis 2014; 32(4):337–44.

25. Levine A, Griffiths A, Markowitz J, et al. Pediatric modification of the Montreal classification for inflammatory bowel disease: the Paris classification. Inflamm Bowel Dis 2011;17(6):1314–21.

26. Cosnes J, Cattan S, Blain A, et al. Long-term evolution of disease behavior of Crohn's disease. Inflamm Bowel Dis 2002;8(4):244–50.

27. Van Limbergen J, Russell RK, Drummond HE, et al. Definition of phenotypic characteristics of childhood-onset inflammatory bowel disease. Gastroenterology 2008;135(4):1114–22.

28. Church PC, Turner D, Feldman BM, et al. Systematic review with meta-analysis: magnetic resonance enterography signs for the detection of inflammation and intestinal damage in Crohn's disease. Aliment Pharmacol Ther 2015;41(2):153–66.

29. Orscheln ES, Dillman JR, Towbin AJ, et al. Penetrating Crohn's disease: does it occur in the absence of stricturing disease? Abdom Radiol (NY) 2018;43(7): 1583–9.

30. Assa A, Amitai M, Greer ML, et al. Perianal pediatric Crohn's disease is associated with a distinct phenotype and greater inflammatory burden. J Pediatr Gastroenterol Nutr 2017;65(3):293–8.

31. Steward MJ, Punwani S, Proctor I, et al. Non-perforating small bowel Crohn's disease assessed by MRI enterography: derivation and histopathological validation of an MR-based activity index. Eur J Radiol 2012;81(9):2080–8.

32. Church PC, Greer MC, Cytter-Kuint R, et al. Magnetic resonance enterography has good inter-rater agreement and diagnostic accuracy for detecting inflammation in pediatric Crohn's disease. Pediatr Radiol 2017;47(5):565–75.

33. Moy MP, Kaplan JL, Moran CJ, et al. MR enterographic findings as biomarkers of mucosal healing in young patients with Crohn's disease. AJR Am J Roentgenol 2016;207(4):896–902.

34. Rimola J, Alvarez-Cofino A, Perez-Jeldres T, et al. Comparison of three magnetic resonance enterography indices for grading activity in Crohn's disease. J Gastroenterol 2017;52(5):585–93.

35. Rimola J, Ordas I, Rodriguez S, et al. Magnetic resonance imaging for evaluation of Crohn's disease: validation of parameters of severity and quantitative index of activity. Inflamm Bowel Dis 2011;17(8): 1759–68.

36. Makanyanga J, Punwani S, Taylor SA. Assessment of wall inflammation and fibrosis in Crohn's disease: value of T1-weighted gadolinium-enhanced MR imaging. Abdom Imaging 2012;37(6):933–43.

37. Hordonneau C, Buisson A, Scanzi J, et al. Diffusion-weighted magnetic resonance imaging in ileocolonic Crohn's disease: validation of quantitative index of activity. Am J Gastroenterol 2014;109(1):89–98.

38. Kim KJ, Lee Y, Park SH, et al. Diffusion-weighted MR enterography for evaluating Crohn's disease: how does it add diagnostically to conventional MR enterography? Inflamm Bowel Dis 2015;21(1):101–9.

39. Bettenworth D, Bokemeyer A, Baker M, et al. Assessment of Crohn's disease-associated small bowel strictures and fibrosis on cross-sectional imaging: a systematic review. Gut 2019;68(6):1115–26.

40. Rieder F, Bettenworth D, Ma C, et al. An expert consensus to standardise definitions, diagnosis and treatment targets for anti-fibrotic stricture therapies in Crohn's disease. Aliment Pharmacol Ther 2018; 48(3):347–57.

41. Lightner AL, Fletcher JG. Duodenal Crohn's disease-a diagnostic conundrum. J Gastrointest Surg 2018; 22(4):761–3.

42. Park SK, Yang SK, Park SH, et al. Long-term prognosis of the jejunal involvement of Crohn's disease. J Clin Gastroenterol 2013;47(5):400–8.

43. Bruining DH, Loftus EV Jr, Ehman EC, et al. Computed tomography enterography detects intestinal wall changes and effects of treatment in patients with Crohn's disease. Clin Gastroenterol Hepatol 2011;9(8):679–83.e1.

44. Peyrin-Biroulet L, Loftus EV Jr, Colombel JF, et al. The natural history of adult Crohn's disease in population-based cohorts. Am J Gastroenterol 2010;105(2):289–97.

45. Faubion WA Jr, Fletcher JG, O'Byrne S, et al. EMerging BiomARKers in Inflammatory Bowel Disease (EMBARK) study identifies fecal calprotectin, serum MMP9, and serum IL-22 as a novel combination of biomarkers for Crohn's disease activity: role of cross-sectional imaging. Am J Gastroenterol 2013; 108(12):1891–900.

46. Mansuri I, Fletcher JG, Bruining DH, et al. Endoscopic skipping of the terminal ileum in pediatric Crohn's disease. AJR Am J Roentgenol 2017; 208(6):W216–24.

47. Samuel S, Bruining DH, Loftus EV Jr, et al. Endoscopic skipping of the distal terminal ileum in Crohn's disease can lead to negative results from ileocolonoscopy. Clin Gastroenterol Hepatol 2012; 10(11):1253–9.

48. Sandborn WJ. Crohn's disease evaluation and treatment: clinical decision tool. Gastroenterology 2014; 147(3):702–5.

49. Bruining DH, Siddiki HA, Fletcher JG, et al. Benefit of computed tomography enterography in Crohn's disease: effects on patient management and physician level of confidence. Inflamm Bowel Dis 2012;18(2): 219–25.

50. Buisson A, Hordonneau C, Goutorbe F, et al. Bowel wall healing assessed using magnetic resonance imaging predicts sustained clinical remission and decreased risk of surgery in Crohn's disease. J Gastroenterol 2019;54(4):312–20.

51. Deepak P, Fletcher JG, Fidler JL, et al. Radiological response is associated with better long-term outcomes and is a potential treatment target in patients with small bowel Crohn's disease. Am J Gastroenterol 2016;111(7):997–1006.

52. Sauer CG, Middleton JP, McCracken C, et al. Magnetic resonance enterography healing and magnetic resonance enterography remission predicts improved outcome in pediatric Crohn's disease. J Pediatr Gastroenterol Nutr 2016;62(3):378–83.

53. Taylor SA, Mallett S, Bhatnagar G, et al. Diagnostic accuracy of magnetic resonance enterography and small bowel ultrasound for the extent and activity of newly diagnosed and relapsed Crohn's disease (METRIC): a multicentre trial. Lancet Gastroenterol Hepatol 2018;3(8):548–58.

Magnetic Resonance in Crohn Disease
Imaging Biomarkers in Assessing Response to Therapy

Jordi Rimola, MD, PhD[a,b,c,*], Nunzia Capozzi, MD[a,d]

KEYWORDS

- Magnetic resonance • Biomarker • Therapeutic response • Crohn disease • Perianal disease

KEY POINTS

- Magnetic resonance (MR) enterography has a key role in both clinical research and practice.
- Using cross-sectional imaging to predict the response to treatment is essential to tailoring treatment.
- Objective and reproducible indexes based on MR findings enable disease severity to be graded, making it possible to assess therapeutic efficacy.
- Pelvic MR imaging is the gold standard for monitoring patients with perianal Crohn disease and helps optimize treatment.

INTRODUCTION

In Crohn disease (CD), the clinical decision making and new drug evaluation processes are based mainly on symptom control. Clinicians order changes to treatment to better manage symptoms associated with inflammatory activity (eg, diarrhea and abdominal pain), impairment of general well-being, or extraintestinal manifestations. The measurements of clinical symptoms alone, for example, by using the Crohn's Disease Activity Index (CDAI), are not a reliable tool, however, to monitor the course if the disease. An analysis of data from the *Study* of Biologic and Immunomodulator Naive Patients in *Crohn Disease (SONIC) trial* showed that 18% of patients classified by the CDAI as having moderate to severe disease (CDAI >220) had no ulcers at endoscopy.[1]

Moreover, after therapeutic intervention, 47% of patients who were classified as in remission by the CDAI (CDAI <150) still had ulcers, and 35% of those whose mucosa had healed were classified as still having active disease.

Imaging, either cross-sectional imaging or endoscopic, has become the standard of care for initial diagnosis of CD and for further follow-up by assessing severity and detecting complications.[2] Clinical symptoms, although relevant for detecting flare-ups of the disease, are subjective, and more objective tools, such as imaging, for detecting active disease are needed.

The therapeutic armamentarium in CD has greatly expanded in the past 2 decades and up to a dozen biologics drugs and immunomodulators are available for modern inflammatory bowel disease (IBD) care.[3] The approach to therapeutics

Disclosure Statement: The authors have nothing to disclose.
[a] Department of Radiology, Hospital Clínic Barcelona, Barcelona, Catalonia, Spain; [b] CIBER-EHD, Barcelona, Catalonia, Spain; [c] University of Barcelona, Barcelona, Catalonia, Spain; [d] Department of Radiology, Hospital S. Orsola-Malpighi, University of Bologna, Via Giuseppe Massarenti, 9, Bologna 40138, Italy
* Corresponding author. Department of Radiology, Hospital Clínic of Barcelona, Carrer de Villarroel 170, Escala 3 Planta 1, Barcelona, Catalonia 08036, Spain.
E-mail address: jrimola@clinic.cat

Magn Reson Imaging Clin N Am 28 (2020) 45–53
https://doi.org/10.1016/j.mric.2019.08.004

has also changed with a more aggressive approach using a treat-to-target philosophy. The most relevant target used in practice and in research is mucosal healing. The healing of ulcerations has been associated with better outcomes in terms of reduction of patient hospitalization and need of surgical resections. Therefore, for guiding therapeutic decisions in patients with CD. it is essential to have accurate and reliable tools to demonstrate healing of inflammatory bowel lesions.

Magnetic resonance enterography (MRE) offers several advantages over other imaging modalities for use in assessing the status of the disease and for the monitorization of CD. MRE enables the assessment of disease activity, which is out of reach of the endoscope (transmural or isolated small bowel disease), which may facilitate the evaluation of the whole small bowel.[4,5] MRE-based assessment might be more responsive to endoscopic activity indices, such as the Simplified Endoscopic Score for Crohn's Disease (SES-CD), which is subject to colonic preparation and technical difficulties.[6] Therefore, in clinical research, for assessment of efficacy outcomes, MRE again ensures assessment of all intestinal segments and avoids operator-dependent variability between baseline and post-treatment assessments. In clinical practice, MRE provides information that changes clinician perspectives and also influences planned therapeutic strategy in a significant proportion of patients.[7] Finally, unlike computed tomography enterography, MRE does not require exposure to ionizing radiation, which is a key aspect considering the general young age at the time of diagnosis and the fact that patients require multiple reassessments of the disease during their life.[2]

In the clinical scenario of perianal fistulizing CD, pelvic magnetic resonance imaging (MRI) has been shown to be a highly accurate noninvasive modality for the diagnosis and classification of perianal fistulas. In addition, pelvic MRI provides detailed information on fistula anatomy, extensions, severity, and presence of perianal collections that is key to planning the best therapeutic approach, usually requiring surgery followed by medical treatment. Currently, pelvic MRI it is considered the gold standard imaging technique for perianal CD.[8]

For the short-term and long-term monitorization of the severity of the disease, in particular in clinical research, the use of quantitative biomarkers allows the conversion of MRE-based observation into a statistically tractable framework. In that regard, the multiparametric nature of MRI has allowed the development of different magnetic resonance (MR)-based indexes using regression models and a valid reference standard. This article reviews the current available biomarkers for measuring the severity of luminal inflammation in CD and discusses the strengths and limitations of each of them. Also, an overview is provided on the scores available for grading the severity of perianal CD based on MRI observations.

INDICES FOR SMALL AND COLON ACTIVITY ASSESSMENT

The derivation of MR-based scores derived from regression models that predict activity assessed by a valid external gold standard (histology or endoscopy) is more stringent than those derived based on expert opinion because only the variables with independent predictor value for severity and activity are selected, whereas those without a proved independent predictor value are excluded from the scoring system. The downside of using tools derived using regression models is that the derived indexes may not be easily applicable in the daily clinical practice if they entail the quantitative measurement of too many or too difficult descriptors.

Magnetic Resonance Index of Activity Score

The MR index of activity (MaRIA)[9] is a composite score that takes into account the bowel wall thickness, relative contrast enhancement on the bowel wall before and after gadolinium injection, presence of ulcers, and presence of mural edema (defined as hyperintensity on T2-weighted sequences). The MaRIA was derived as a simplified score to quantify disease activity from MRE findings in each segment of the terminal ileum or the colon:

MaRIAseg = (1.5 × wall thickness) + (0.02 × relative contrast enhancement) + (5 × edema) + (10 × ulcers at MRE)

where wall thickness is measured in millimeters at the thickest point in the segment; edema and ulcer are each assigned a value of 1, when there is evidence of either in the segment (or 0 when not). RCE represents the relative contrast enhancement of the intestinal wall between pregadolinium and postgadolinium T1-weighted sequences, where

RCE = (mean of 3 region of interest [ROI] measurements postgadolinium − mean of 3 ROI measurements pregadolinium)/mean of 3 ROI measurements before gadolinium

The global MaRIA score provides information at patient level and is computed as the sum total of the subscores of each intestinal segment.[9,10]

The MaRIA score provides a continuous and quantitative index of inflammation severity that has been applied in different studies and currently is the best characterized score to grade disease activity using MRE.[11] Two cutoffs were selected in a cross-validation study using ileocolonoscopy as gold standard, a MaRIA subscore of greater than or equal to 7 for depicting segments with active disease (received operating characteristic [ROC] area under the curve [AUC] = 0.933; sensitivity 0.87 and specificity 0.87) and a subscore greater than or equal to 11 units for identifying segments with severe disease activity (ROC AUC = 0.965; sensitivity 0.92 and specificity 0.92).[9,10] Moreover, the MaRIA was devised to be highly concordant with the objective endoscopic score, the SES-CD, in the deep small bowel intestine.[12] For these reasons, including through the contribution of the MRE in detecting CD complications, such as strictures, fistula, and abscess, this index can be used as prognostic biomarker to select and assess patient for inclusion in clinical trials.[13]

Besides diagnostic accuracy and responsiveness, reproducibility is a critical property of an evaluative instrument, especially when serial measurements are required. In this sense, the MaRIA has shown almost perfect intrarater reproducibility when was read by central readers, supporting its use as a reliable tool in drug development trials.[11,13,14]

The MaRIA score was used to determine the responsiveness of MRE after induction treatment in CD patients after medical therapeutic intervention (after either corticoids or tumor necrosis factor [TNF] inhibitors), showing that the MaRIA score at segment level is sensitive for detecting healing after medical intervention and reliable in detecting the persistence of ulcerations (overall accuracy of 90% for detecting endoscopic mucosal healing)[15,16] (**Table 1**).

These observations were externally validated by other groups.[17–19] In a similar study, Stoppino and colleagues[17] reported on observations of global MaRIA change in response to anti-TNF at week 26 in a cohort of 27 patients with CD and suggest that the optimal cutoff point for identification of patients who had achieved mucosal healing at week 26 was 30.8. In contrast to the original global MaRIA, including 6 segments, in the work of Stoppino and colleagues, global MaRIA was scored as the summation of only 5 segments. This disagreement, however, may be a point of attention suggesting that more stringent criteria for detecting remission at patient level should be used. In that regard, for patients to be in remission, all segmental MaRIA scores must be less than 7.

Overall, these results indicate that the MaRIA index can be used for the monitorization of changes over time.

More recently, a Japanese group[19] explored the diagnostic yield of the MaRIA score for detecting healing of lesions in the small bowel using enteroscopy as a reference standard, reporting a similar and high accuracy in both the terminal ileum and in the proximal segments of the small bowel (see **Table 1**).

Despite the wide use of the MaRIA score, the authors acknowledge this index has some limitations. The main drawback is that normal bowel segments contribute to the global MaRIA score whereas ideally normal segments should be scored as zero. As a consequence, in patients with resected segments, an underestimation of the global score occurs. Regarding the acceptance for its calculation, although it takes into account only 4 items, its computation requires measurement of different quantitative parameters (wall thickness and relative contrast enhancement), which is, as a result, time consuming because it must be calculated segment by segment. Hence, a simpler MR tool with faster assessment for measuring disease activity in CD, called simplified MaRIA,[16] has been recently released and further validation in independent cohorts is still required (**Fig. 1**).

Diffusion-weighted Imaging, Apparent Diffusion Coefficient, and the Clermont Score

The Clermont score (or diffusion-weighted imaging [DWI]-MaRIA) is similar to the MaRIA index, but it uses the apparent diffusion coefficient (ADC) value, calculated by means of the DWI sequence, instead of relative contrast enhancement. To derive and validate the DWI-MaRIA score, the same MRE (by means of the MaRIA score) was considered the reference standard, resulting a new index where wall thickness, mural edema, and ulcerations are included as independent predictors for activity, together with the ADC.[20,21] The formula to calculate the segmental activity according to Clermont score is as follows:

Clermont score = (1.646 × wall thickness) + (−1.321 × ADC) + (5.613 × edema) + (8.306 × ulcers at MRE) + 5.039

A Clermont subscore of greater than or equal to 8.4 is indicative of bowel segments with active CD, and a subscore of greater than or equal to 12.5 units identifies segments with moderate to severe CD activity, with ulcers at endoscopy. As expected, a close correlation had been found

Table 1
Evidence supporting the use of magnetic resonance index of activity as a biomarker for monitorization of activity

Context of Use/Characterization	Publication	Comments/Evidence
MRE and definition of score and patient selection	Rimola et al,[9] 2009	Derivation of the MaRIA score highly correlated to CDEIS/endoscopy
	Rimola et al,[10] 2011	Validation of the MaRIA correlation with CDEIS/endoscopy
	Takenaka et al,[12] 2015	High concordance between MaRIA and SES-CD; MaRIA accurate at detecting inflammatory activity in small bowel proximal to terminal ileum
Therapeutic response assessment	Ordás et al,[15] 2014	Concordance between MRE and endoscopy assessment of response to TNF inhibitors and corticosteroids in the terminal ileum and colon
	Stoppino et al,[17] 2016	Concordance between MRE and endoscopy assessment of response to TNF inhibitors in the terminal ileum and colon
	Takenaka et al,[19] 2018	Concordance between MRE and enteroscopy assessment of response to TNF inhibitors in the small bowel
Prognosis	Buisson et al,[18] 2017	Achieving transmural healing according to MaRIA score was associated with longer period in corticosteroid-free remission ($P = .0001$) and no needed surgery within 2 y ($P = .0332$)
Reproducibility	Tielbeek et al,[14] 2013	Inter-reader reliability
	Coimbra et al,[13] 2016	Test-retest, intrareader, and inter-reader reliability
	Jairath et al,[11] 2018	Test-retest, intrareader, and inter-reader reliability

between both MaRIA and Clermont indexes,[20] almost perfect (r = 0.99) in the terminal ileum but lower in the colon.

Regarding the responsiveness of Clermont index after induction treatment in CD patients, MRE remission predicted mucosal healing with specificity of 79.4% and negative predictive value of 84.4%, according to Clermont criteria (no segmental Clermont score >12.5)[18] (**Table 2**).

Because Clermont score mirrors the MaRIA score, it has the same previously mentioned limitations, but, at this time, no simplified version is under investigation. In addition, the main specific limitation for the Clermont score is its applicability due to the current lack of standardized method for DWI acquisition, including technical parameters and bowel preparation.[22] An additional limitation is the inherent difficulty to measure ADC in normal-appearing thin intestinal wall. Lastly, the

lack of standardization of DWI acquisition and interplatform MR variability in the calculation of ADC values may represent a source of variability and may hamper its use in large-scale trails.[23]

Bowel Motility as Biomarker

As is already known, segments with active inflammation present a reduced motility compared with noninflamed segments.[24,25] Although MRI-derived bowel motility quantification is now feasible, motility itself has yet to be validated as a biomarker of inflammation in CD, and the available literature is currently limited.

MRE-measured motility has a significant negative correlation with endoscopic and histopathologic severity of inflammation (the greater the inflammatory burden, the larger the reduction in motility).[25] An additional attractive approach in

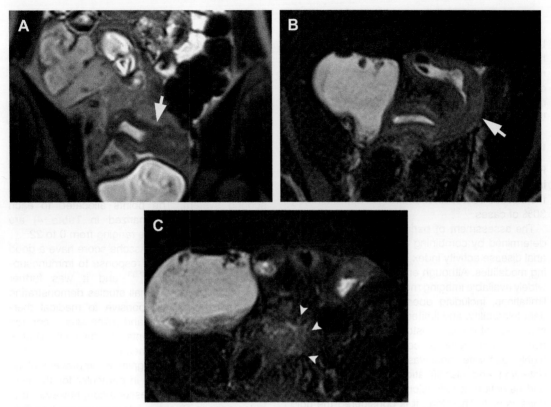

Fig. 1. (*A*) Coronal T2-weighted imaging of the terminal ileum shows segmental thickening of the intestine wall (*arrow*). (*B*) Axial T2-weighted with fat saturation of the same segment shows hypersignal intensity of the same segment, indicating the presence of edema (*arrow*) and (*C*) perienteric fat stranding on regional mesenteric fat (*arrowheads*). No convincing findings of ulcers were seen on this segment. The segmental simplified MaRIA score accounts for 3 points.

using motility as quantitative biomarker for monitoring inflammation is the lack of the use of intravenous contrast agents. Sequences can be acquired by repletion of breath holds during 20 seconds, focused on pathologic segments, and acquiring 1 image/second using T2-weighted coronal images. Currently, however, these sequences remain optional, according to literature[26]; further efforts are needed in order to standardize the acquisition and even the radiological interpretation that is still subjective or requires a specific dedicated commercial software.

Table 2
Evidence supporting the use of diffusion-weighted imaging, apparent diffusion coefficient, and Clermont score as biomarkers for monitorization of activity

Context of Use/Characterization	Publication	Comments/Evidence
MRE and definition of score and patient selection	Hordonneau et al,[20] 2014	MRE, including DWI, is a reliable tool to assess bowel inflammation in colonic (ADC) and ileal (Clermont score) CD
Therapeutic response assessment	Buisson et al,[18] 2017	MaRIA and Clermont scores were equally adequate in detecting endoscopic ulcer healing on endoscopy with high specificity. Sensitivity and positive predictive values were moderate.

The main existing concerns are regarding whether or not other histologic subtracts in the bowel, such as fibrosis deposition, also may have an impact on motility impairment and regarding determining standard values that would differentiate segments with active disease from remission regardless its location in the small bowel.

BIOMARKERS FOR PERIANAL DISEASE

Perianal lesions are common and occur in approximately 20% of patients suffering with CD along the disease course and recurring in approximately 30% of cases.[27,28]

The assessment of perianal disease activity is determined by combining clinical symptom (perianal disease activity index) and findings on imaging modalities. Although endoanal ultrasound is a widely available imaging modality, it has important limitations, including operator dependency, patient tolerability, and limited scope for a complete evaluation of complex fistulas and collections far from the anal canal. By contrast, pelvic MRI is a highly accurate noninvasive modality for the detection and classification of perianal fistulas and detection of extensions and perianal collections as well. Therefore, it is considered the gold standard imaging technique for perianal CD.[8,29]

Compared with luminal CD, there are few indexes that can be used as biomarkers for perianal CD monitorization.

Van Assche Index

The best-characterized index to assess perianal disease based on MR is the Van Assche index (VAI). It was originally developed to meet the need for a standardized tool that could measure response of perianal fistulizing CD to medical therapy[30] and avoid patients serving as their own controls to determine improvement or worsening of perianal disease[31] (Table 3).

VAI combines the anatomic fistula characteristics with MRI findings linked to the inflammation and has a total of 6 descriptors, including, number, anatomic classification of the fistulas, extension, collections, T2 signal intensity of the main tract, and rectal wall involvement. When multiple fistulas coexist, the fistula with the highest severity (most predominant) is assessed using the Van Assche scoring system. The points allocated to each assessment (as summarized in Table 4) are summed to a total score ranging from 0 to 22.

Changes in the Van Assche score have a good correlation with clinical response to immunosuppressant treatment[30,32,33] and it was further partially validated in small studies demonstrating that this score is responsive to medical therapy.[34,35] Savoye-Collet and colleagues[36] reported that in a cohort of patients with perianal CD after 1 year of infliximab therapy, clinical response was associated with significant improvement on the Van Assche score, in particular for the item T2 hyperintensity. The assumption, however, that a decrease in T2 signal intensity implies less fluid content and, therefore, less active inflammation has not been validated.

One major caveat for implementing this index as an endpoint in clinical trials is the lack of a cutoff point for defining fistula healing that ideally should be zero.[30] Another limitation of this index is that the responsiveness of each individual item of the score was not determined, representing still relevant unmet needs, because this information may

---

Table 3
Evidence supporting the use of pelvic magnetic resonance imaging to monitor perianal fistulizing disease activity

Context of Use/Characterization	Publication	Comments/Evidence
MRI for grading and monitoring perianal fistulizing CD	Van Assche et al,[30] 2003	Development of an MRI-based score of perianal CD severity to assess the anatomic evolution of Crohn fistulas. Partial validation of Van Assche score
Pelvic MRI may guide treatment in CD perianal fistulas	Ng et al,[34] 2009	Once MRI healing has occurred (hypoenhancement and hyposignal on T2), perianal fistulas remain healed, while remaining on or stopping anti-TNF α therapy.
Attempt to improve Van Assche score	Samaan et al,[38] 2017	Modification of Van Assche score. MR descriptors were selected based on inter-rater reliability.

Table 4
Van Assche score and modified Van Assche score descriptors—item weights in parentheses

Descriptor	Van Assche Score	Modified Van Assche Score
Number of fistula tracts	None (0) Single, unbranched (1) Single, branched (2) Multiple (3)	None (0) Single, unbranched (1) Single, branched (2) Multiple (3)
Location (according to Parks system)	Extrasphincteric or intersphincteric (1) Transsphincteric (2) Suprasphincteric (3)	Submucosal (0) Intersphincteric (1) Transsphincteric (2) Extrasphincteric (3) Suprasphincteric (4)
Extensions	Infralevatoric (1) Supralevatoric (2)	Absent (0) Infralevatoric (1) Horseshoe (2) Supralevatoric (3)
Hyperintensity on T2	Absent (0) Mild (4) Pronounced (8)	Absent (0) Mild (1) Pronounced (2)
Collections (cavities >3-mm diameter)	Absent (0) Present (4)	—
Rectal wall involvement	Normal (0) Thickened (2)	Normal (0) Thickened (1) Increased signal intensity (2)
Inflammatory mass	—	Absent (0) Diffuse (1) Focal (2) Collection—small (3–10 mm) (3) Collection—medium (11–20 mm) (4) Collection large (>20 mm) (5)
Dominant feature of primary tract and extensions	—	Predominantly fibrous (0) Predominantly filled by granulation tissue (1) Predominantly filled by fluid or pus (2)

Adapted from Samaan MA, Puylaert CAJ, Levesque BG, et al. The development of a magnetic resonance imaging index for fistulising Crohn's disease. Aliment Pharmacol Ther 2017;46(5):516-528; with permission.

be key to developing a more robust index for assessing fistula healing.[37]

Modified Van Assche Index

The modified VAI is a novel tool for grading the severity of fistulizing CD developed in attempt to improve the original VAI. A panel of experts in imaging of perianal disease identified and excluded the VAI descriptors with suboptimal reliability and endorsed other new items with higher inter-rater performance.[38] As result, the modified VAI contains 7 descriptors, including number of fistula, location, extension, hyperintensity on T2-weighted images, rectal wall involvement, inflammatory mass, and dominant feature of primary tract and extension (see **Table 4**). Additionally, to improve

communication, the same panel of experts is developing standardized definitions through a systematic consensus process.

Although this index has not yet been applied in therapeutic intervention trials, the main advantage over the original VAI is its higher reproducibility.[38] The responsiveness of the new index, however, which would require comparing pretreatment and post-treatment MRIs in patients receiving a treatment of known efficacy, remains unclear, and also pending is establishing the minimally significant score change for response and cutoff for remission.

FUTURE DIRECTIONS AND CONCLUSIONS

Due to the increasing importance of mucosal healing as a measure of treatment success and the likelihood of maintaining long-term remission, endoscopic indices are now favored over clinical indices. The inherent limitations of ileo-colonoscopy for assessing the right colon, in particular the terminal ileum, especially in the setting of severe inflammation involving this segment, and considerations that both clinical symptoms and endoscopy are not sensitive to ruling out the presence of penetrating complications in CD represent the current drawbacks for its use in clinical trials. Because MRE assessment is highly concordant with endoscopy for assessing bowel inflammation and has a higher ability to detect penetrating disease that also is beneficial for patients, it will provide a better assessment of risk-to-benefit ratio for enrolling in clinical trials.[13] Currently, MRE alone is intended to be used as objective assessment. Although scarce, recent evidence shows that transmural healing assessed by MRE is associated with improved long-term outcomes in CD and may be a more suitable target than mucosal endoscopic healing. If confirmed in further studies, the added value of MRE as a prognostic biomarker will reinforce the role of MRE as modality for evaluating treatment efficacy in clinical trials and research.

Effective drug therapy for prevention and treatment of CD-associated strictures is an unmet need, but uncertainties regarding diagnostic methods and definitions have hampered the clinical development of antifibrotic compounds for stricturing CD.[39] There are a few potential drugs that have been approved for pulmonary fibrosis but, to date, there have been no clinical trials of antifibrotics in CD.[40,41] Developing a reliable and responsive index for MRE evaluation of fibrostenotic CD is a research priority.[42] This will enable integration of imaging findings in a systematic and reproducible manner. A validated tool for quantifying stricturing CD also will be crucial for clinical trial development in this field, both as an inclusion criterion and as an outcome measure.

REFERENCES

1. Peyrin-Biroulet L, Reinisch W, Colombel J-F, et al. Clinical disease activity, C-reactive protein normalisation and mucosal healing in Crohn's disease in the SONIC trial. Gut 2014;63(1):88–95.

2. Maaser C, Sturm A, Vavricka SR, et al. ECCO guideline/consensus paper ECCO-ESGAR guideline for diagnostic assessment in IBD part 1: initial diagnosis, monitoring of known IBD, detection of complications. J Crohns Colitis 2018;1–32. https://doi.org/10.1093/ecco-jcc/jjy113.

3. Panés J, Salas A. Past, present and future of therapeutic interventions targeting leukocyte trafficking in inflammatory bowel disease. J Crohns Colitis 2018; 12(Suppl_2):633–40.

4. Jauregui-Amezaga A, Rimola J, Ordás I, et al. Value of endoscopy and MRI for predicting intestinal surgery in patients with Crohn's disease in the era of biologics. Gut 2015;64(9):1397–402.

5. Faubion WA, Fletcher JG, Byrne SO, et al. EMerging BiomARKers in Inflammatory Bowel Disease (EMBARK) study identifies fecal calprotectin, serum MMP9, and Serum IL-22 as a novel combination of biomarkers for Crohn's disease activity: role of cross-sectional imaging. Am J Gastroenterol 2013;108:1891–900.

6. Jairath V, Levesque BG, Vande Casteele N, et al. Evolving concepts in phases i and ii drug development for crohn's disease. J Crohns Colitis 2017; 11(2). https://doi.org/10.1093/ecco-jcc/jjw137.

7. García-Bosch O, Ordás I, Aceituno M, et al. Comparison of diagnostic accuracy and impact of MRI and colonoscopy for the management of Crohn's disease. J Crohns Colitis 2016;10(6):663–9.

8. Gecse KB, Bemelman W, Kamm MA, et al. A global consensus on the classification, diagnosis and multidisciplinary treatment of perianal fistulising Crohn's disease. Gut 2014;63(9):1381–92.

9. Rimola J, Rodriguez S, García-Bosch O, et al. Magnetic resonance for assessment of disease activity and severity in ileocolonic Crohn's disease. Gut 2009;58(8):1113–20.

10. Rimola J, Ordás I, Rodriguez S, et al. Magnetic resonance imaging for evaluation of Crohn's disease: validation of parameters of severity and quantitative index of activity. Inflamm Bowel Dis 2011;17(8). https://doi.org/10.1002/ibd.21551.

11. Jairath V, Ordas I, Zou G, et al. Reliability of measuring ileo-colonic disease activity in crohn's disease by magnetic resonance enterography. Inflamm Bowel Dis 2018;24(2):440–9.

12. Takenaka K, Ohtsuka K, Kitazume Y, et al. Correlation of the endoscopic and magnetic resonance scoring systems in the deep small intestine in Crohn's disease. Inflamm Bowel Dis 2015;21(8): 1832–8.

13. Coimbra AJF, Rimola J, O'Byrne S, et al. Magnetic resonance enterography is feasible and reliable in multicenter clinical trials in patients with Crohn's disease, and may help select subjects with active inflammation. Aliment Pharmacol Ther 2016;43(1): 61–72.

14. Tielbeek JAW, Makanyanga JC, Bipat S, et al. Grading crohn disease activity with MRI: interobserver variability of MRI features, MRI scoring of severity, and correlation with crohn disease endoscopic index of severity. Am J Roentgenol 2013; 201(6):1220–8.

15. Ordás I, Rimola J, Rodríguez S, et al. Accuracy of magnetic resonance enterography in assessing response

to therapy and mucosal healing in patients with crohn's disease. Gastroenterology 2014;146(2):374–82.

16. Ordás I, Rimola J, Alfaro I, et al. Development and validation of a simplified magnetic resonance index of activity for crohn's disease. Gastroenterology 2019. https://doi.org/10.1053/j.gastro.2019.03.051.

17. Stoppino LP, Della Valle N, Rizzi S, et al. Magnetic resonance enterography changes after antibody to tumor necrosis factor (anti-TNF) alpha therapy in Crohn's disease: correlation with SES-CD and clinical-biological markers. BMC Med Imaging 2016;16(1):1–9.

18. Buisson A, Pereira B, Goutte M, et al. Magnetic resonance index of activity (MaRIA) and Clermont score are highly and equally effective MRI indices in detecting mucosal healing in Crohn's disease. Dig Liver Dis 2017;49(11):1211–7.

19. Takenaka K, Ohtsuka K, Kitazume Y, et al. Utility of magnetic resonance enterography for small bowel endoscopic healing in patients with crohn's disease. Am J Gastroenterol 2018;113(2):283–94.

20. Hordonneau C, Buisson A, Scanzi J, et al. Diffusion-weighted magnetic resonance imaging in ileocolonic Crohn's disease: validation of quantitative index of activity. Am J Gastroenterol 2014;109(1):89–98.

21. Buisson A, Hordonneau C, Goutte M, et al. Diffusion-weighted magnetic resonance entero-colonography is highly effective to detect ileocolonic endoscopic ulcerations in crohn's disease. Aliment Pharmacol Ther 2015;42(4):452–60.

22. Dohan A, Taylor S, Hoeffel C, et al. Diffusion-weighted MRI in Crohn's disease: current status and recommendations. J Magn Reson Imaging 2016;44:1381–96.

23. Rimola J, Alvarez-Cofiño A, Pérez-Jeldres T, et al. Comparison of three magnetic resonance enterography indices for grading activity in Crohn's disease. J Gastroenterol 2017;52(5):585–93.

24. Froehlich JM, Waldherr C, Stoupis C, et al. MR motility imaging in Crohn's disease improves lesion detection compared with standard MR imaging. Eur Radiol 2010;20(8):1945–51.

25. Menys A, Atkinson D, Odille F, et al. Quantified terminal ileal motility during MR enterography as a potential biomarker of Crohn's disease activity: a preliminary study. Eur Radiol 2012;22(11):2494–501.

26. Taylor SA, Avni F, Cronin CG, et al. The first joint ESGAR/ESPR consensus statement on the technical performance of cross-sectional small bowel and colonic imaging. Eur Radiol 2017;27(6):2570–82.

27. Schwartz DA, Loftus EV, Tremaine WJ, et al. The natural history of fistulizing Crohn's disease in Olmsted County, Minnesota. Gastroenterology 2002;122(4):875–80.

28. Eglinton TW, Barclay ML, Gearry RB, et al. The spectrum of perianal crohn's disease in a population-based cohort. Dis Colon Rectum 2012;55:773–7.

29. Sheedy SP, Bruining DH, Dozois EJ, et al. MR imaging of perianal Crohn disease. Radiology 2017; 282(3):628–45.

30. Van Assche G, Vanbeckevoort D, Bielen D, et al. Magnetic resonance imaging of the effects of infliximab on perianal fistulizing Crohn's disease. Am J Gastroenterol 2003;98(2):332–9.

31. Bell S, Williams A, Wiesel P, et al. The clinical course of fistulating Crohn's disease. Aliment Pharmacol Ther 2003;17(9):1145–51.

32. Horsthuis K, Lavini C, Bipat S, et al. Perianal Crohn disease: evaluation of dynamic contrast-enhanced MR Imaging as an Indicator of disease activity. Radiology 2009;251(2):380–7.

33. Karmiris K, Bielen D, Vanbeckevoort D, et al. Long-term monitoring of infliximab therapy for perianal fistulizing Crohn's disease by using magnetic resonance imaging. Clin Gastroenterol Hepatol 2011; 9(2):130–6.

34. Ng SC, Plamondon S, Gupta A, et al. Prospective evaluation of anti-tumor necrosis factor therapy guided by magnetic resonance imaging for Crohn's perineal fistulas. Am J Gastroenterol 2009;104(12): 2973–86.

35. Horsthuis K, Ziech MLW, Bipat S, et al. Evaluation of an MRI-based score of disease activity in perianal fistulizing Crohn's disease. Clin Imaging 2011;35(5):360–5.

36. Savoye-Collet C, Savoye G, Koning E, et al. Fistulizing perianal Crohn's disease: contrast-enhanced magnetic resonance imaging assessment at 1 year on maintenance anti-TNF-alpha therapy. Inflamm Bowel Dis 2011;17(8):1751–8.

37. Panés J, Rimola J. Perianal fistulizing Crohn's disease: pathogenesis, diagnosis and therapy. Nat Rev Gastroenterol Hepatol 2017;14(11): 652–64.

38. Samaan MA, Puylaert CAJ, Levesque BG, et al. The development of a magnetic resonance imaging index for fistulising Crohn's disease. Aliment Pharmacol Ther 2017;46(5):516–28.

39. Rieder F, Fiocchi C, Rogler G. Mechanisms, management, and treatment of fibrosis in patients with inflammatory bowel diseases. Gastroenterology 2017;152(2):340–50.e6.

40. King TE, Bradford WZ, Castro-Bernardini S, et al. A phase 3 trial of pirfenidone in patients with idiopathic pulmonary fibrosis. N Engl J Med 2014; 370(22):2083–92.

41. Richeldi L, du Bois RM, Raghu G, et al. Efficacy and safety of nintedanib in idiopathic pulmonary fibrosis. N Engl J Med 2014;370(22):2071–82.

42. Rieder F, Bettenworth D, Ma C, et al. An expert consensus to standardise definitions, diagnosis and treatment targets for anti-fibrotic stricture therapies in Crohn's disease. Aliment Pharmacol Ther 2018;48:347–57.

Malabsorption Syndromes, Vasculitis, and Other Uncommon Diseases

Daniel A. Adamo, MD[a], Shannon P. Sheedy, MD[a], Christine O. Menias, MD[b], Michael L. Wells, MD[a], Jeff L. Fidler, MD[a,*]

KEYWORDS

- MR enterography • Small intestine • Inflammation • Malabsorption • Vasculitis

KEY POINTS

- MR enterography plays a major role in the evaluation of patients with suspected small bowel disease and can be extremely helpful in guiding the next most appropriate step in the workup of patients.
- MR enterography may be able to diagnose clinically unsuspected small bowel disorders.
- Many diseases involving the small bowel produce nonspecific findings such as wall thickening and mural hyperenhancement.
- Radiologist familiarity with clinical aspects of small bowel diseases, small bowel and associated imaging findings, and potential complications is imperative to construct an accurate differential diagnosis.

INTRODUCTION

MR enterography (MRE) is frequently ordered for patients with suspected small bowel disorders. The most common indication is for the diagnosis and surveillance of Crohn disease, but many other diseases can involve the small bowel. Patients with suspected small bowel disease may present with abdominal pain, nausea, vomiting, diarrhea, gastrointestinal tract bleeding, and malabsorption prompting small bowel imaging. However, many patients may present with vague or nonspecific abdominal symptoms and MRE may be ordered to screen the entire abdomen including the small bowel. In this latter scenario, MRE may be able to diagnose clinically unsuspected small bowel disorders.

In this article, diseases causing malabsorption, vasculitides, and some of the less common small bowel diseases are reviewed. Space restrictions preclude an in-depth discussion of these entities; however, several excellent review articles are referenced for further reading. The clinical presentations, diagnostic criteria, and imaging findings of these diseases are discussed. Because the imaging findings in several small bowel diseases is nonspecific and/or overlap, radiologists must correlate clinical data with imaging to develop a narrower differential diagnosis. The unique or characteristic findings in certain diseases are also emphasized.

ETIOLOGIES

Several classification schemes have been derived for diseases of the small bowel, including based on underlying histopathology (**Box 1**); however, because of the complexity of these diseases, significant overlap exists.

Disclosure Statement: No disclosures.
a Department of Radiology, Mayo Clinic, 200 First Street Southwest, Rochester, MN 55902, USA; b Department of Radiology, Mayo Clinic, 5777 East Mayo Boulevard, Phoenix, AZ 85054, USA
* Corresponding author. Department of Radiology, Mayo Clinic, 200 First Street Southwest, Rochester, MN 55905.
E-mail address: fidler.jeff@mayo.edu

Magn Reson Imaging Clin N Am 28 (2020) 55–73
https://doi.org/10.1016/j.mric.2019.09.001

Box 1
Etiologies of small bowel diseases producing multiple areas or long segments of bowel wall thickening

Edema and impaired drainage
  Ischemia
  Angioedema
  Hypoproteinemia
  Cirrhosis
  Lymphangiectasis
  Venous obstruction
Infection
  Campylobacter
  Yersinia
  Salmonella
  Giardiasis
  Tuberculosis/mycobacterium avium infection
  Clostridium difficile
  Cryptosporidiosis
  Cytomegalovirus
  Whipple disease
Hemorrhage
  Spontaneous
  Ischemia
  Trauma
  Vasculitis
  Amyloid
Inflammation
  Nonsteroidal anti-inflammatory drug enteropathy
  Radiation
  Chemotherapy
  Vasculitis
  Immune mediated (Crohn disease, CeD, autoimmune, graft-versus-host disease)
  Peritonitis
Infiltrative conditions
  Amyloid
  Eosinophilic gastroenteritis
  Mastocytosis
Fibrosis
  Crohn disease
  Eosinophilic gastroenteritis
  Amyloid
  Radiation

◀ Post-inflammatory
Neoplastic and cancer-related treatment
  Lymphoma
  Multifocal neuroendocrine
  Metastases
  Radiation
  Chemotherapy-induced conditions
  Graft-versus-host disease

APPROACH TO BOWEL WALL THICKENING

Many diseases involving the small bowel produce nonspecific findings such as wall thickening and mural hyperenhancement. Under-distension can mimic pathologic bowel wall thickening, resulting in false-positive interpretations and unnecessary workup and treatment. Because MR obtains multiple sequences over the course of the examination, the radiologist has the opportunity to assess peristalsis and various degrees of distension over time and to determine whether suspected areas of wall thickening persist or resolves with improved distension.

The list of potential etiologies involving the small bowel can be overwhelming and, when encountering a case with bowel wall thickening in clinical practice, it can be difficult to construct a refined differential diagnosis. Several approaches have been proposed, including a pattern-based approach to computed tomography (CT) scans,[1] which can be translated for use with MRE. This approach evaluates the enhancement characteristics (degree/pattern); the degree, length, and symmetry of the bowel wall thickening; the segmental location of involvement; and any associated abnormalities. If using this approach with MRE, one must be aware that MRE is more sensitive to contrast enhancement and mild inflammation than is CT scanning and that mild inflammation may coexist in areas of fibrosis; this can result in a more stratified enhancement pattern on MR imaging in entities that typically seem to be more homogenous appearance on CT scans. An alternate approach uses a checklist of specific diseases that can be reviewed to determine if the imaging findings are consistent. Whichever approach is used, radiologist familiarity with the clinical aspects of these diseases as well as with small bowel and associated imaging findings and potential complications is imperative.

GUIDANCE OF PATIENT WORKUP

In many cases, imaging may not be able to determine a specific diagnosis, but can be extremely helpful in guiding the next most appropriate step in the workup of patients. Therefore, an accurate and concise differential diagnosis is critical. For example, laboratory testing may be appropriate for some patients (eg, suspected infection, ischemia, angioedema and celiac disease [CeD]). In other patients, imaging may be most helpful to guide endoscopic evaluation and biopsy (eg, suspected CeD, eosinophilic gastroenteritis, Crohn disease, and neoplasm). Notably, endoscopic evaluation is often negative and not helpful in submucosal disease processes, such as angioedema. Prompt referral to surgery for cases of suspected ischemia or definitive neoplasm can be aided by imaging. In benign self-limited etiologies, such and angioedema and infection, serial follow-up can be suggested for assessing the resolution of findings and excluding a chronic process that may need further evaluation.

CELIAC DISEASE

CeD is an immune-mediated enteropathy caused by gluten exposure in genetically susceptible individuals. The classic symptoms of steatorrhea, weight loss, pain, and failure to thrive are only seen in approximately one-third of individuals. Other presenting symptoms include iron deficiency anemia, premature osteoporosis, infertility, dermatitis herpetiformis, and miscellaneous conditions (dental abnormalities, arthritis, hyposplenism, selective IgA deficiency). A delay in diagnosis is common in patients with nonspecific or atypical symptoms; in these patients, imaging may be the first to suggest the diagnosis.

Screening for CeD can be performed using a celiac serology cascade. The definitive diagnosis is made with upper endoscopy and biopsy with clinical and histologic response to a gluten-free diet. The characteristic histologic changes are those of villous atrophy; however, this finding is nonspecific and can be seen with other disorders. Crypt hyperplasia and increased T lymphocytes are also present.

The imaging findings of CeD have been extensively reported.[2] Many findings are nonspecific, but when seen can suggest the diagnosis and further workup. One of the earliest signs is small bowel dilatation (**Fig. 1**) and increased small bowel fluid owing to both hypersecretion and malabsorption. Mild fold and wall thickening may be present secondary to decreased albumin, hypersecretion, inflammation, or superimposed complication (discussed elsewhere in this article). The reversal of the small bowel fold pattern is the most specific finding, but is often absent. Initially there is a decrease in the jejunal fold pattern (see **Fig. 1**) with subsequent increase in ileal folds termed "jejunization." The duodenum may have a featureless appearance and submucosal fat may be present in the duodenum and proximal jejunum. Transient intussusceptions occur secondary to the dilated, atonic bowel and altered peristalsis (**Fig. 2**). Multiple small mesenteric nodes are frequently present secondary to the chronic inflammation. Several other signs have also been reported.[2]

Patients with known CeD who present with persistent or recurrent signs and symptoms and with villous atrophy despite more than 12 months of adherence to a gluten-free diet are considered to have refractory celiac. Refractory CeD is classified as type I or type II. Type II refractory CeD demonstrates clonal T-cell receptor rearrangement and abnormal immunophenotype of intraepithelial cells[3]; these patients have an increased prevalence of ulcerative jejunoileitis (UJ) and enteropathy-associated T-cell

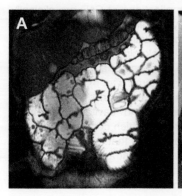
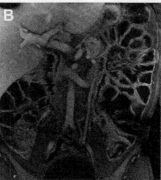

Fig. 1. CeD. A 35-year-old man presents with diarrhea and abdominal pain. (*A*) Coronal fast imaging employing steady-state acquisition and (*B*) coronal T1-weighted postcontrast MRE images demonstrate a malabsorption pattern with diffuse small bowel dilatation and a decrease in the normal jejunal fold pattern.

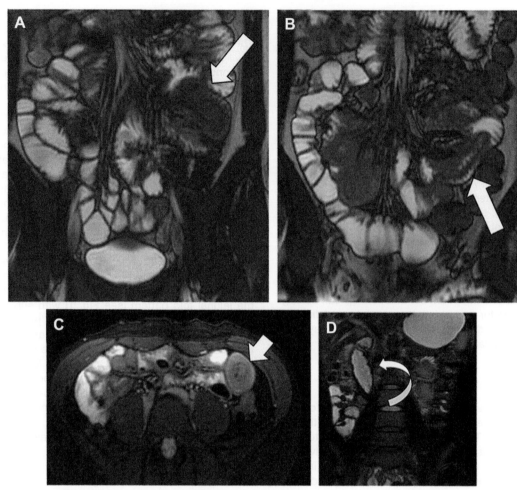

Fig. 2. CeD with enteroenteric intussusceptions. A 19-year-old woman with a previous history of intussusception treated conservatively now presents with abdominal bloating and nausea. (*A, B*) Coronal T2-weighted images and (*C*) axial T2-weighted image from an MRE demonstrate multifocal small bowel intussusceptions (*white arrows* in *A–C*). (*D*) Coronal T2-weighted image shows loss of the duodenal fold pattern (*curved white arrow*). Subsequent endoscopy showed flat-appearing duodenal mucosa. Duodenal biopsy demonstrated malabsorption pattern with total villous atrophy, crypt hyperplasia, and surface epithelial degeneration with increased intraepithelial lymphocytes, highly suggestive of celiac sprue. (*Adapted from* [*B, C*] Sheedy SP, Barlow JM, Fletcher JG, et al. Beyond moulage sign and TTG levels: the role of cross-sectional imaging in celiac sprue. Abdom Radiol (NY) 2017;42(2):370; with permission.)

lymphoma. Patients with UJ present with fever, pain, distension, and weight loss.[3] UJ occurs in up to 70% of patients with type II refractory CeD and is preneoplastic with up to 50% developing enteropathy-associated T-cell lymphoma.

MRE is helpful in evaluating patients with suspected refractory CeD. MRE can demonstrate resolution of findings in healed CeD and can detect bowel abnormalities, such as wall thickening, mural hyperenhancement, and mesenteric stranding or edema suggesting UJ (**Fig. 3**). Given the variable distension of the jejunum on MRE, some prefer MR enteroclysis to improve jejunal

distension[4] if complications of CeD are clinically suspected. It may be difficult to differentiate UJ from lymphoma on imaging as both can present with areas of wall thickening and hyperenhancement (**Fig. 4**). The presence of a more focal mass is suggestive of lymphoma (**Fig. 5**).

Other complications that can develop in CeD include hyposplenism and cavitary mesenteric lymph node syndrome, which consist of lipid-rich hyaline-filled lymph nodes that have fat signal intensity and may demonstrate fat–fluid levels (**Fig. 6**). These conditions usually occur in patients with severe uncontrolled CeD.

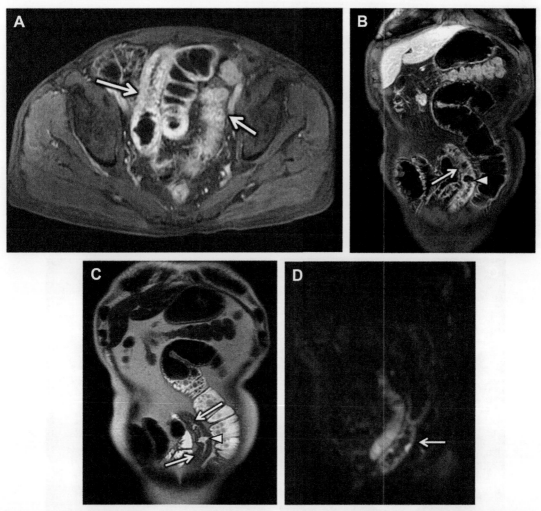

Fig. 3. Refractory CeD with UJ. A 58-year-old man with history of refractory CeD who presented with a 6-month history of persistent abdominal pain, diarrhea, and recent hospitalization for small bowel obstruction. (*A*) Coronal and (*B*) axial T1-weighted postcontrast MRE images, and (*C*) coronal T2-weighted MRE image demonstrate wall thickening and mural hyperenhancement (*arrows*) with mucosal ulceration (*arrowhead*) in a loop of mid small bowel causing proximal dilatation. (*D*) Diffusion-weighted image demonstrates associated restricted diffusion (*arrow*) in the affected bowel loops. Surgical pathology demonstrated moderate active jejunitis with pseudopyloric metaplasia and ulceration.

WHIPPLE DISEASE

Whipple disease is a rare multisystem disease, more common in middle-aged white males, which can involve the small bowel, heart valves, central nervous system, and joints. Potential bowel symptoms include weight loss, diarrhea (secondary to malabsorption), cramps, anorexia, and occasionally gastrointestinal bleeding.[5,6] Whipple disease is caused by an infection with *Tropheryma whipplei*, which responds to antibiotic therapy; however, Whipple disease can be difficult to diagnose because of the atypical presenting symptoms.

Without treatment, Whipple disease is ultimately fatal and even with treatment relapse occurs in up to 33%.[6] The infection leads to a disorder in bacterial disposal resulting in macrophages with bacteria and abnormal lipid accumulation. This results in classically described lipid-laden periodic acid-Schiff–positive staining macrophages on histology.[5,6]

The imaging findings include dilatation secondary to malabsorption and diffuse or patchy micronodules located in the proximal small bowel. However, because of the inferior spatial resolution of MRE compared with fluoroscopic barium

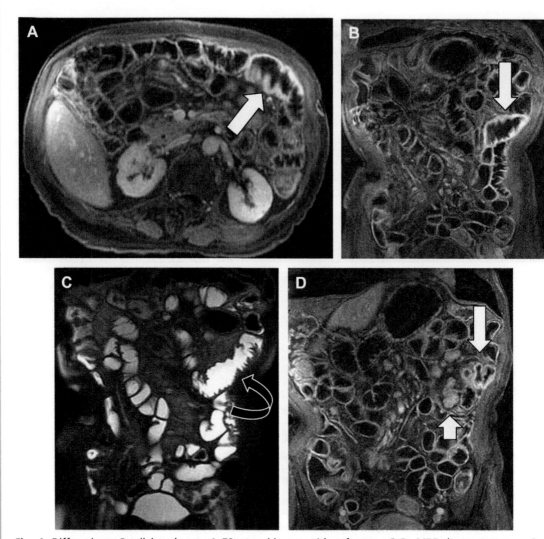

Fig. 4. Diffuse large B-cell lymphoma. A 79-year-old man with refractory CeD. MRE demonstrates an 8-cm segment of abnormal appearing jejunum in the left upper quadrant with wall thickening and hyperenhancement. (*A, B*) Postcontrast T1-weighted images with fat suppression (*straight arrows* in A, B, and D) with (*C*) blunted and thickened folds (T2-weighted coronal image, *curved arrow*) and (*D*) many enlarged mesenteric lymph nodes (postcontrast image, *short arrow*). Double balloon endoscopy and biopsy was consistent with diffuse large B-cell lymphoma. B-cell lymphoma is an unusual complication of CeD, but it does occur. (*From* Sheedy SP, Barlow JM, Fletcher JG, et al. Beyond moulage sign and TTG levels: the role of cross-sectional imaging in celiac sprue. Abdom Radiol (NY) 2017;42(2):382; with permission.)

examinations, this nodularity is usually not appreciated. On MRE, there may be bowel wall and fold thickening and the folds may appear somewhat nodular or bulbous (**Fig. 7**). A unique association is the presence of fat-containing mesenteric lymph nodes.

EOSINOPHILIC GASTROENTERITIS

Eosinophilic gastroenteritis is rare and, thus, it is difficult to estimate the incidence. Eosinophilic gastroenteritis usually occurs in the fourth and fifth decades of life with a slight male predominance.[7] Patients usually have a history of allergic disorders and may have certain food intolerances. Abdominal pain, nausea, and vomiting are the most frequent symptoms. The diagnosis requires the presence of gastrointestinal symptoms, a mucosal eosinophilic infiltrate on biopsy, or an imaging study showing findings consistent with eosinophilic gastroenteritis with associated clinical peripheral eosinophilia in the absence of other

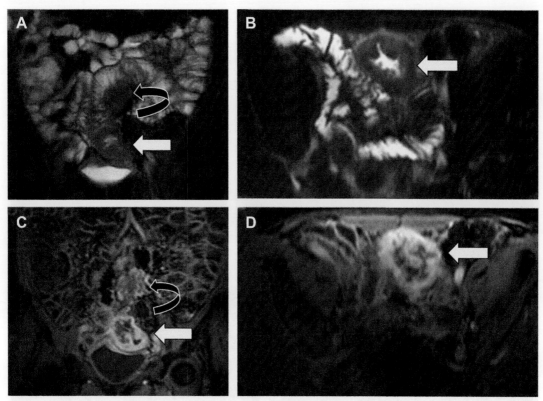

Fig. 5. Multifocal enteropathy associated T-cell lymphoma of the jejunum. (*A*) Coronal and (*B*) axial T2-weighted images with fat saturation and (*C, D*) coronal and axial postcontrast images demonstrate a 6-cm enhancing, centrally necrotic distal jejunal mass in the pelvis (*straight white arrows*) without obstruction and with associated lymphadenopathy (*curved black arrows*). Segmental resections of small bowel were performed, revealing multifocal enteropathy-associated T-cell non-Hodgkin's lymphoma. (*From* [*B, C*] Sheedy SP, Barlow JM, Fletcher JG, et al. Beyond moulage sign and TTG levels: the role of cross-sectional imaging in celiac sprue. Abdom Radiol (NY) 2017;42(2):380; with permission.)

known causes of eosinophilia (eg, drug reaction, parasitic infection, malignancy). Treatment includes dietary adjustment with or without steroids, which may be combined with other immunosuppressive drugs. Surgery may be required in obstructive cases.

The 3 forms of eosinophilic gastroenteritis are classified by the layer of the bowel wall involved.[7] Usually 2 of the 3 types coexist. The imaging findings depend on the layer of the bowel wall that is involved.[8] The mucosal form is most common and leads to mucosal inflammation and ulcerations. Patients present with pain, diarrhea, and bleeding. Imaging findings include the presence of wall thickening, edema, and hyperenhancement consistent with inflammation (**Fig. 8**). The muscularis form is the second most common type and causes muscle thickening, which is seen on imaging as mural thickening with luminal narrowing and strictures that can lead to obstruction. A full-thickness biopsy is required to definitively confirm

the muscularis form of eosinophilic gastroenteritis. The degree of wall hyperenhancement depends on the amount of associated inflammation. The serosal form is the least common form. On imaging, there may be serosal thickening with intense serosal enhancement and ascites is typically seen. Peripheral eosinophilia is also commonly present with this form.

BOWEL ISCHEMIA

Small bowel ischemia can result from arterial occlusion, venous occlusion, low flow states and with bowel obstruction. Patients typically present with acute abdominal pain and are usually evaluated with CT scans. However, mesenteric venous thrombosis or occlusion (not uncommon to see in inflammatory bowel disease patients) may present more gradually with nonspecific abdominal pain; therefore, these patients may be referred for MRE. Venous ischemia typically produces more

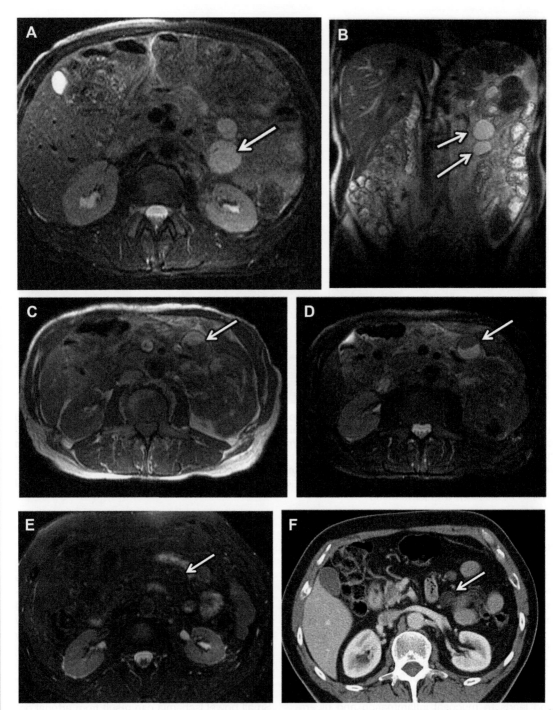

Fig. 6. Cavitary mesenteric lymph node syndrome. A 62-year-old man with known CeD and a 5-month history of weight loss, nausea, and anorexia. (*A*) Axial and (*B*) coronal T2-weighted MRE images with fat suppression demonstrate multiple cystic masses (*arrows*) within the mesenteric fat. Two years later, (*C*) axial T1-weighted and (*D*) axial T2-weighted image with fat suppression MR images demonstrate development of fat–fluid levels in the lymph nodes. (*E*) Subsequent axial-T2 weighted image with fat suppression and (*F*) contrast-enhanced axial CT images from 3 years later demonstrate complete fatty replacement of the lymph nodes (*arrows*). (*From* [*D*] Sheedy SP, Barlow JM, Fletcher JG, et al. Beyond moulage sign and TTG levels: the role of cross-sectional imaging in celiac sprue. Abdom Radiol (NY) 2017;42(2):385; with permission.)

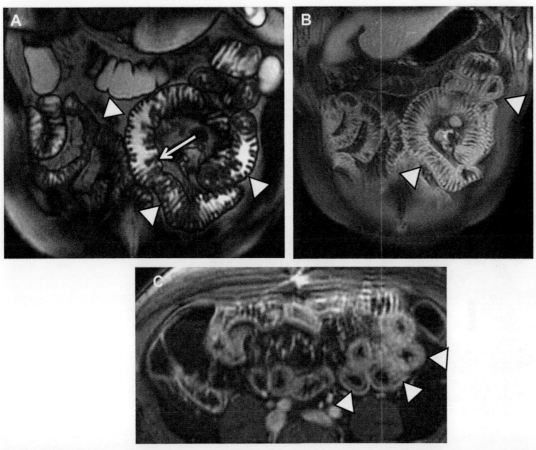

Fig. 7. Whipple disease. A 45-year-old man presented with weight loss, diarrhea, and fevers. (*A*) Coronal fast imaging employing steady-state acquisition, (*B*) coronal, and (*C*) axial T1-weighted postcontrast MRE images demonstrate diffuse small bowel dilatation with diffuse fold thickening (*arrowheads*), which seems to be nodular (*arrow*) in some locations. Duodenal biopsy showed histiocytes containing periodic acid-Schiff–positive, diastase resistant material, and was positive on polymerase chain reaction for *Tropheryma whipplei*.

bowel wall thickening and edema than the other forms of ischemia (**Fig. 9**). The development of mesenteric venous collaterals may lead to some decompression of the venous obstruction. Development of small bowel varices can be a source of gastrointestinal bleeding.

ANGIOEDEMA

Angioedema is caused by a defect in the complement activation system. This can be secondary to a C1 esterase deficiency or inhibitors of the angiotensin-converting enzyme and/or receptors. These defects lead to an unchecked complement activation system with subsequent development of vasodilatation and increased capillary permeability. The C1 esterase inhibitor deficiency can be hereditary (subclassified into 3 forms: those with low levels, those with low

function, and estrogen dependent) or acquired. Angiotensin-converting enzyme inhibitors, which are frequently used for hypertension, may incite angioedema and can occur days or years after initiating the drug.

Angioedema is edema involving the deep dermis, subcutaneous tissues, or submucosa. Patients may present with angioedema involving the skin, airways, or bowel. Patients with bowel involvement typically present with acute abdominal pain. Imaging findings consist of marked bowel wall thickening, submucosal edema, and ascites (**Fig. 10**).[9,10] Ischemia may be of concern given the acute presentation and mural edema. Correlation with laboratory tests and the clinical history of angiotensin-converting enzyme inhibitor receptor medications helps to suggest the diagnosis. Not infrequently these patients may present with recurring episodes of acute

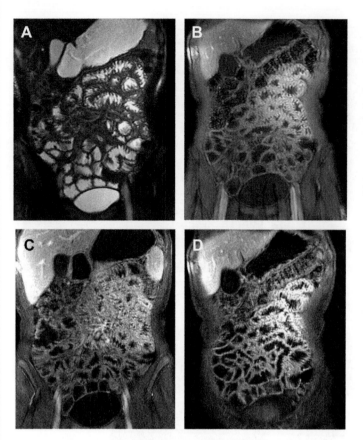

Fig. 8. Eosinophilic gastroenteritis. A 32-year-old man with a multiyear history of diarrhea and recent bloody stools. (*A*) Coronal T2-weighted image with fat suppression and (*B–D*) post-contrast coronal T1-weighted MRE images demonstrate diffuse thickening of the wall and folds affecting the entire small bowel with mild mural hyperenhancement. Endoscopic biopsy demonstrated eosinophilic infiltration consistent with eosinophilic gastroenteritis. The fold thickening, lack of ascites, and positive biopsy suggests this represents the mucosal form of the disease.

abdominal pain with bowel wall thickening that resolves quickly. Angioedema should be considered in this scenario because more chronic inflammatory diseases such as Crohn disease should not resolve, nor do they present with such mural edema. A vasculitis (discussed elsewhere in this article) can also present with recurrent episodes of acute abdominal pain and similar mural edema and may be difficult to differentiate, although the degree of thickening may be greater with angioedema.

AMYLOIDOSIS

Amyloidosis is a rare protein deposition disease and is classified based on the precursor protein. Light chain amyloidosis is the most common type in the United States; it is a plasma cell dyscrasia and is linked to multiple myeloma. AA amyloidosis (secondary amyloidosis) results as a complication of chronic inflammatory diseases such as rheumatoid arthritis and Crohn disease. The hereditary form is rare. Other forms include dialysis-related, age-related, and organ-specific amyloid.[11–13]

Gastrointestinal amyloid deposition may be associated with systemic involvement (80%–98%) or isolated (20%).[11,12] It is more common with AA amyloidosis than with light chain amyloidosis[14,15] and most commonly affects the small bowel.[12] In the small bowel, it can be diffuse or can be deposited focally resulting in a mass-like appearance or amyloidoma (**Fig. 11**).[13,16]

The clinical manifestations and imaging findings depend on which portion of the bowel wall is involved. Deposition around the terminal vessels can lead to edema, inflammation, ischemia, hemorrhage and ulceration. Neuromuscular deposition can lead to muscular atrophy and dysmotility, resulting in bowel dilatation (pseudo-obstruction). Deposition in the mucosa or submucosa leads to ulcers, bleeding, and malabsorption. The appearance of the wall and fold thickening varies depending on the presence of inflammation, hemorrhage, or fibrosis. Fold thickening may be polypoid,[11–13] and in the distal small bowel can lead to jejunization of the ileum.[11,16] Strictures may result from subsequent development of fibrosis. The mural deposition may give the bowel a rigid appearance with separation of the bowel loops. There may be

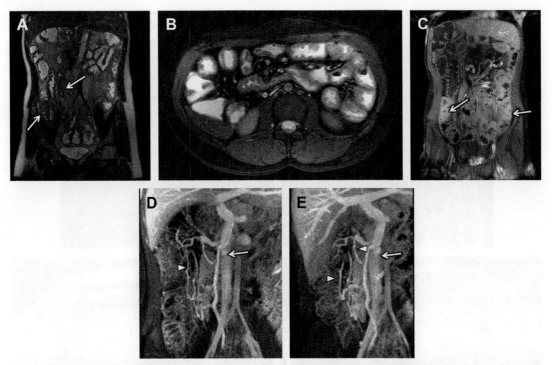

Fig. 9. Chronic venous ischemia. A 21-year-old woman with a history of gastroschisis with intestinal malrotation, and surgical history of pylorus-sparing Whipple pancreaticoduodenectomy for solid pseudopapillary epithelial neoplasm of the pancreas presents with chronic abdominal pain. (*A*) Coronal T2-weighted image, (*B*) axial fast imaging employing steady-state acquisition image with fat suppression, and (*C*) coronal postcontrast T1-weighted image with fat suppression demonstrate diffuse wall and fold thickening of the jejunum and ileum (*arrows*). (*D, E*) Coronal postcontrast T1-weighted maximum intensity projection images show occlusion of the superior mesenteric vein (*arrows*) with multiple venous collaterals (*arrowheads*). If adequate collateral flow is developed, there may be less bowel wall thickening and symptoms. Because of persistent symptoms, a superior mesenteric vein stent was placed (not shown).

soft tissue thickening in the mesentery secondary to amyloid infiltration.[12,17]

SYSTEMIC SCLEROSIS

Systemic sclerosis or scleroderma is a connective tissue disease that affects the skin, blood vessels, and internal organs, including the gastrointestinal tract. The small bowel is involved in approximately 40% to 90% of patients.[18] Deposition of collagen in the wall of the bowel leads to a vasculitis, telangectasias, and submucosal fibrosis. The changes can extend into the muscularis and cause muscle atrophy. Patients may be asymptomatic, or have malabsorption secondary to bacterial overgrowth, pain, diarrhea, and pseudo-obstruction.

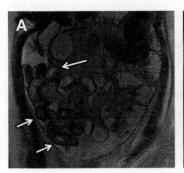

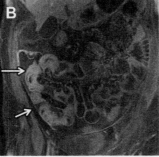

Fig. 10. Angioedema. A 52-year-old woman presented with acute abdominal pain. (*A*) Coronal T2-weighted single shot fast spin echo and (*B*) coronal postcontrast T1-weighted MRE images demonstrate bowel wall thickening in the ileum (*arrows*). The bowel wall thickening demonstrates high T2 signal and stratified enhancement consistent with submucosal edema. Also note the presence of ascites. The patient had recently started an angiotensin-converting enzyme inhibitor for hypertension.

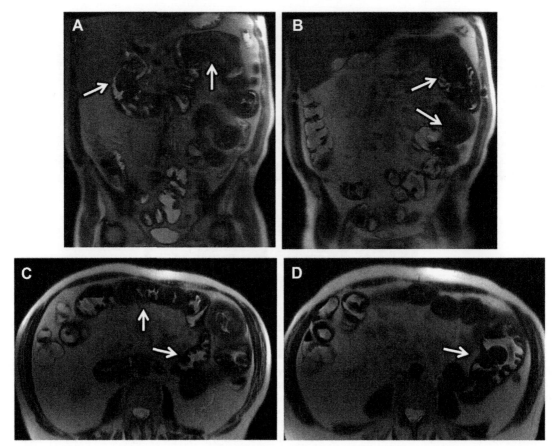

Fig. 11. Amyloidosis. A 65-year-old man with known amyloid presents with abdominal pain and gastrointestinal bleeding. (*A, B*) Coronal and (*C, D*) axial T2-weighted single shot fast spin echo MRE images demonstrate multiple low T2 signal areas of bowel wall and fold thickening in the duodenum and small bowel (*arrows*). Several of these areas seem to be more nodular and mass-like. Biopsy of a duodenal lesion showed findings consistent with amyloid.

Imaging findings include dilated small bowel, mainly proximally. A hide-bound appearance can occur with dilatation of the small bowel and crowding of the folds owing to smooth muscle atrophy and fibrosis of the inner circular layer of the tunica muscularis combined with longitudinal smooth muscle contraction[19] (**Fig. 12**). Other findings include large broad-mouthed the

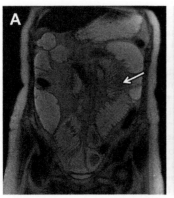 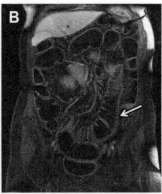

Fig. 12. Scleroderma. A 62-year-old woman with known history of scleroderma presented with a 90-pound weight loss. (*A*) Coronal T2-weighted MRE image and (*B*) coronal postcontrast T1-weighted MRE image demonstrate dilated loops of small bowel with closely space folds producing the classic hide-bound appearance of the folds in the jejunum (*arrows*).

sacculations occur on the mesenteric border not the antimesenteric border of the bowel wall secondary to submucosal fibrosis and pneumatosis cystoides intestinalis.

NONSTEROIDAL ANTI-INFLAMMATORY DRUG ENTEROPATHY

Nonsteroidal anti-inflammatory drugs are commonly used drugs that can lead to complications in the small bowel ranging from ulcerations to diaphragm-like strictures. Patients may present with intermittent episodes of small bowel obstruction and occult gastrointestinal bleeding. The typical imaging findings include multiple circumferential, short, or focal ring-like strictures that are in close proximity and are usually located in the ileum.[20] Frequently, there is some associated active inflammation that leads to mural hyperenhancement and helps to improve detection (**Fig. 13**). These may findings be frequently overlooked as contractions if they are predominately fibrotic or not causing obstruction. Focal symmetric diaphragm-like strictures are nonspecific and can also be seen in Crohn disease and a rare condition, cryptogenic multifocal ulcerative and stenosing enteritis.[21]

VASCULITIS

Classification of vasculitis is based on vessel size and can be primary or secondary (**Box 2**).[22,23] Primary vasculitides consist of large vessel (aorta and branches), medium vessel (visceral artery and branches), or small vessel (intraparenchymal) disease, and variable or Behçets disease.[22–25] Secondary vasculitides include those associated with systemic disease such as systemic lupus erythematosus, long standing rheumatoid arthritis, and sarcoid.[26,27] The most common vasculitides that involve the small bowel include immunoglobulin A vasculitis (Henoch-Schoenlein purpura), antineutrophil cytoplasmic autoantibody-associated vasculitis, polyarteritis nodosa, and Behçets disease. Vasculitides are associated with inflammatory leukocytes in the walls of the vessel, which can lead ischemia. Patients with small bowel involvement often present with acute abdominal pain, nausea, vomiting, diarrhea, and gastrointestinal bleeding. The imaging findings include bowel wall thickening with submucosal edema, ischemia, and hemorrhage (**Figs. 14** and **15**). Perforation and strictures can also develop. Ischemic changes occurring at unusual sites, in patients without

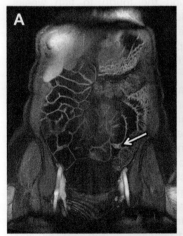
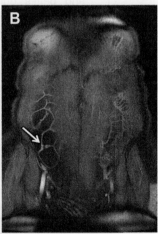
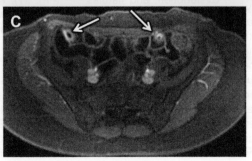

Fig. 13. Nonsteroidal anti-inflammatory drug (NSAID) enteropathy. A 64-year-old woman with a history of recurrent partial small bowel obstructions and chronic NSAID use for low back pain. (*A, B*) Coronal and (*C*) axial postcontrast T1-weighted MRE images demonstrate multiple focal short diaphragmatic strictures in the ileum with mild mural hyperenhancement (*arrows*), and associated mild dilation of proximal loops of small bowel. Subsequent surgical resection demonstrated moderately active ileitis with ulceration, stricture, and diaphragm formation consistent with a clinical history of NSAID use.

risk factors or of younger age, the history of one of the associated conditions, and other organ involvement should suggest the diagnosis of vasculitis.[28] Because many of the vasculitides that involve the small bowel affect the smaller vessels, it is difficult to see vascular changes on the MR image, which are best demonstrated on conventional angiography. However, occasionally aneurysms, vascular wall thickening, or irregularity may be seen with the medium vessel vasculitides.[28] The imaging findings of intestinal Behçets disease may be similar to Crohn disease. Behçets disease usually has larger ulcerations and 1 study showed that a polypoid appearance and more homogenous mural enhancement pattern was seen more frequent in Behçets disease, whereas strictures, long segment disease, and the

involvement of more proximal ileal loops favored Crohn disease.[24]

JEJUNOILEAL DIVERTICULOSIS

Small bowel diverticulosis is an acquired condition that occurs most commonly in the jejunum. Because of stasis within the diverticula, patients can develop bacterial overgrowth and present with abdominal pain, diarrhea, and malabsorption. Other complications include diverticulitis, bleeding, pseudo-obstruction, perforation, and chronic pneumoperitoneum.[29] This condition is frequently overlooked on cross-sectional imaging studies because the diverticula are mistaken as fluid-filled bowel. The appearance of featureless bowel without the normal jejunal fold pattern and a barely perceptible wall in the region of the jejunum should suggest diverticulosis (**Fig. 16**).

MALIGNANCY-ASSOCIATED CONDITIONS
Radiation-Induced Small Bowel Disease

Pelvic radiation is commonly performed for a variety of pelvic malignancies. Radiation-induced small bowel disease can be subdivided into acute and chronic forms.[30] The acute form occurs during or shortly after a course of radiation usually during the second week and peaks during the fourth to fifth weeks. Symptoms include colicky abdominal pain, bloating, nausea, diarrhea, and gastrointestinal bleeding. The process is usually self-limiting and resolves within 3 months.[30] In the acute form, there is arteriolar obliteration, which leads to edema, inflammation, and ischemic-like changes. Imaging findings included wall thickening, luminal narrowing, and stratified hyperenhancement.[31,32] The chronic form usually occurs 18 months to 6 years after radiation therapy.[30] Symptoms include pain, intermittent small bowel obstruction, bloating, diarrhea, steatorrhea, and malabsorption. Imaging findings include strictures, which may have superimposed inflammation, bowel dilatation from dysfunction, and fistulas[31,32] (**Fig. 17**). Findings are most commonly seen where the bowel is in a fixed location, such as the terminal ileum or areas of adhesions.

Graft-Versus-Host Disease

Graft-versus-host disease (GVHD) can present after allogeneic hematopoietic stem cell transplantation with an incidence of up to 59% and usually involves the skin, gastrointestinal tract, and liver.[33] Patients may present with nausea,

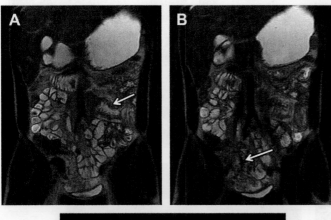

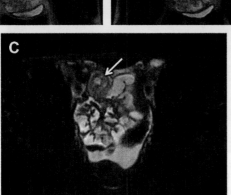

Fig. 14. Vasculitis. A 21-year-old man presented with a 2-month history of abdominal pain and diffuse maculopapular skin rash affecting the entire body. (*A*) Coronal T2-weighted MRE image demonstrates mural thickening in the proximal jejunum (*arrow*). (*B*) Coronal T2-weighted MRE image and (*C*) axial fast imaging employing steady-state acquisition with fat suppression MRE image show mural thickening and edema in the terminal ileum (*arrows*) with associated ascites. The patient was initially treated for Crohn disease, however, subsequent biopsy demonstrated findings most consistent with a small vessel vasculitis.

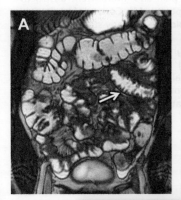

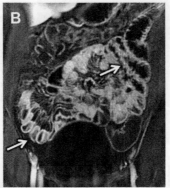

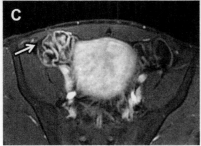

Fig. 15. Vasculitis. A 21-year-old man with history of episodic abdominal pain and bowel wall thickening on CT scan. Prior resection of the jejunum showed changes of a necrotizing vasculitis. Cutaneous biopsy showed changes of IgA vasculitis. MRE performed during an episode of abdominal pain demonstrates subtle areas of wall and fold thickening (*arrows*) and mild hyperenhancement on (*A*) coronal fast imaging employing steady-state acquisition, (*B*) coronal, and (*C*) axial postcontrast MRE images.

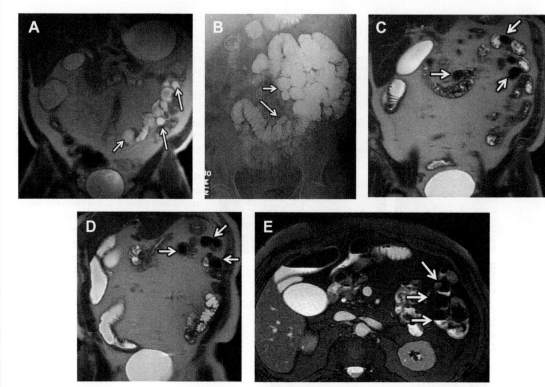

Fig. 16. Jejunoileal diverticulosis. (*A–E*) Two separate patients with jejunoileal diverticulosis. (*A*) Coronal T2-weighted MRE image shows multiple featureless fluid-filled outpouchings in the jejunum (*arrows*). (*B*) Corresponding image from a small bowel series shows multiple jejunal diverticula (*arrows*). (*C*) Coronal and (*D*) axial T2-weighted MRE images, and (*E*) axial fast imaging employing steady-state acquisition with fat suppression MRE image demonstrate multiple thin-walled air-filled jejunal diverticula.

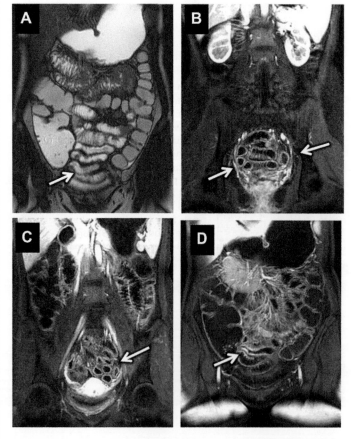

Fig. 17. Radiation-induced small bowel disease. A 60-year-old woman with a prior history of radiation for gynecologic malignancy presents with abdominal pain and intermittent obstructive symptoms. (*A*) Coronal fast imaging employing steady-state acquisition and (*B–D*) coronal postcontrast T1-weighted MRE images demonstrate long segments of wall thickening, mural hyperenhancement, and luminal narrowing (*arrows*) consistent with radiation-induced small bowel disease.

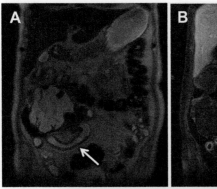
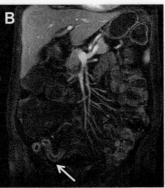
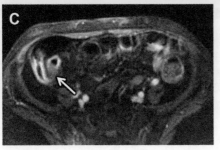

Fig. 18. Late-onset acute GVHD. A 64-year-old woman with prior allogeneic bone marrow transplantation for chronic lymphocytic leukemia. Ten months after transplantation, she presented with diarrhea and gastrointestinal bleeding. (*A*) Coronal T2-weighted, (*B*) coronal, and (*C*) axial postcontrast T1-weighted MRE images demonstrate a long segment of wall thickening, stratified mural hyperenhancement, and luminal narrowing (*arrows*). Subsequent colonoscopy and biopsy showed changes consistent with GVHD.

vomiting, and profuse diarrhea with gastrointestinal involvement. GVHD can be classified as acute, presenting up to 100 days after transplantation, late-onset acute GVHD, chronic, or overlap.[33] Gastrointestinal findings without skin involvement may be seen in up to 20% of cases. Acute GVHD imaging findings include bowel wall thickening, submucosal edema, and stratified hyperenhancement (**Fig. 18**). The presence of diffuse involvement of the small bowel and associated colonic involvement helps to differentiate the imaging findings from other complications, such as infection and neutropenic colitis. As the folds become denuded, the bowel becomes featureless. In chronic GVHD, bowel wall thickening, luminal narrowing, strictures, and webs can occur (**Fig. 19**). The featureless fold pattern combined with long segments of luminal narrowing produces the classic ribbon bowel appearance.

Chemotherapy-Induced Disorders

Because the use of new targeted chemotherapies, including monoclonal antibodies and small molecular inhibitors, is increasing, new side effects involving the gastrointestinal tract are being recognized, including venous thrombosis, bowel ischemia, and tumoral or gastrointestinal bleeding. A unique disorder that has been identified with tyrosine kinase inhibitors is the development of impaired lymphatic drainage, which leads to lymphangiectasis within the bowel wall. This lymphangiectasis occurs as numerous focal small fat signal

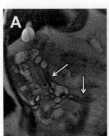
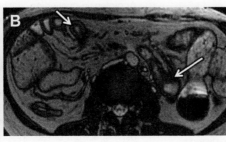

Fig. 19. Chronic GVHD. A 38-year-old woman who underwent allogeneic stem cell transplantation and developed acute GVHD involving the skin and gastrointestinal tract with diarrhea. Three years later, she presented with abdominal pain. (*A*) Coronal T2-weighted and (*B*) axial fast imaging employing steady-state acquisition MRE images show long segments of wall thickening and luminal narrowing (*arrows*) consistent with strictures from chronic GVHD.

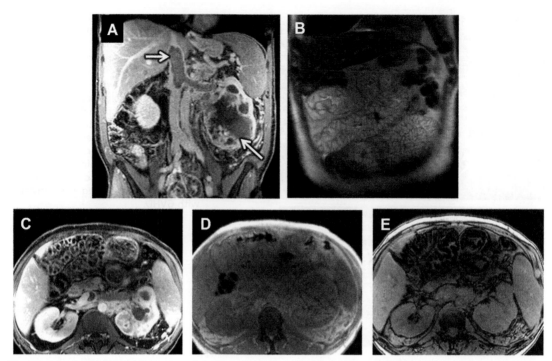

Fig. 20. Tyrosine kinase inhibitor-associated lymphangiectasis. (*A*) A 46-year-old man receiving a tyrosine kinase inhibitor for metastatic renal cell carcinoma extending into the inferior vena cava (*arrows*). There are innumerable small round collections in the small bowel that have fat signal intensity on all sequences including (*B*) coronal T2-weighted, (*C*) axial postcontrast T1-weighted images, and (*D*) axial in-phase and (*E*) out-of-phase images.

intensity collections within the bowel wall[34] (**Fig. 20**).

SUMMARY

Many diseases can involve the small bowel and produce wall thickening and inflammation. In this article we have reviewed some of the less common disorders, which may lead to malabsorption and other gastrointestinal symptoms. Awareness of these less commonly encountered conditions is important to help construct an accurate differential diagnoses and drive more appropriate clinical management.

REFERENCES

1. Macari M, Megibow AJ, Balthazar EJ. A pattern approach to the abnormal small bowel: observations at MDCT and CT enterography. AJR Am J Roentgenol 2007;188(5):1344–55.
2. Sheedy SP, Barlow JM, Fletcher JG, et al. Beyond moulage sign and TTG levels: the role of cross-sectional imaging in celiac sprue. Abdom Radiol (NY) 2017;42(2):361–88.
3. Al-Bawardy B, Barlow JM, Vasconcelos RN, et al. Cross-sectional imaging in refractory celiac disease. Abdom Radiol (NY) 2017;42(2):389–95.
4. Van Weyenberg SJ, Meijerink MR, Jacobs MA, et al. MR enteroclysis in refractory celiac disease: proposal and validation of a severity scoring system. Radiology 2011;259(1):151–61.
5. Bures J, Kopacova M, Douda T, et al. Whipple's disease: our own experience and review of the literature. Gastroenterol Res Pract 2013;2013:478349.
6. Fenollar F, Puechal X, Raoult D. Whipple's disease. N Engl J Med 2007;356(1):55–66.
7. Zhang M, Li Y. Eosinophilic gastroenteritis: a state-of-the-art review. J Gastroenterol Hepatol 2017; 32(1):64–72.
8. Anuradha C, Mittal R, Yacob M, et al. Eosinophilic disorders of the gastrointestinal tract: imaging features. Diagn Interv Radiol 2012;18(2):183–8.
9. Scheirey CD, Scholz FJ, Shortsleeve MJ, et al. Angiotensin-converting enzyme inhibitor-induced small-bowel angioedema: clinical and imaging findings in 20 patients. AJR Am J Roentgenol 2011; 197(2):393–8.
10. Vallurupalli K, Coakley KJ. MDCT features of angiotensin-converting enzyme inhibitor-induced visceral angioedema. AJR Am J Roentgenol 2011;196(4): W405–11.
11. Kim SH, Han JK, Lee KH, et al. Abdominal amyloidosis: spectrum of radiological findings. Clin Radiol 2003;58(8):610–20.

12. Ozcan HN, Haliloglu M, Sokmensuer C, et al. Imaging for abdominal involvement in amyloidosis. Diagn Interv Radiol 2017;23(4):282–5.

13. Georgiades CS, Neyman EG, Barish MA, et al. Amyloidosis: review and CT manifestations. Radiographics 2004;24(2):405–16.

14. Menke DM, Kyle RA, Fleming CR, et al. Symptomatic gastric amyloidosis in patients with primary systemic amyloidosis. Mayo Clin Proc 1993;68(8):763–7.

15. Okuda Y, Takasugi K, Oyama T, et al. Amyloidosis in rheumatoid arthritis–clinical study of 124 histologically proven cases. Ryumachi 1994;34(6):939–46 [in Japanese].

16. Mainenti PP, Segreto S, Mancini M, et al. Intestinal amyloidosis: two cases with different patterns of clinical and imaging presentation. World J Gastroenterol 2010;16(20):2566–70.

17. Araoz PA, Batts KP, MacCarty RL. Amyloidosis of the alimentary canal: radiologic-pathologic correlation of CT findings. Abdom Imaging 2000;25(1):38–44.

18. Nagaraja V, McMahan ZH, Getzug T, et al. Management of gastrointestinal involvement in scleroderma. Curr Treatm Opt Rheumatol 2015;1(1):82–105.

19. Pickhardt PJ. The "hide-bound" bowel sign. Radiology 1999;213(3):837–8.

20. Frye JM, Hansel SL, Dolan SG, et al. NSAID enteropathy: appearance at CT and MR enterography in the age of multi-modality imaging and treatment. Abdom Imaging 2015;40(5):1011–25.

21. Singh A, Sahu MJ, Panigrahi MK, et al. Cryptogenic multifocal ulcerous stenosing enteritis (CMUSE): a tale of three decades. ACG Case Rep J 2017;4:e44.

22. Watts RA, Robson J. Introduction, epidemiology and classification of vasculitis. Best Pract Res Clin Rheumatol 2018;32(1):3–20.

23. Jennette JC. Overview of the 2012 revised International Chapel Hill Consensus Conference nomenclature of vasculitides. Clin Exp Nephrol 2013;17(5):603–6.

24. Peker E, Erden A, Erden I, et al. Intestinal Behcet disease: evaluation with MR enterography-A case-control study. AJR Am J Roentgenol 2018;211(4):767–75.

25. Mahr A, de Menthon M. Classification and classification criteria for vasculitis: achievements, limitations and prospects. Curr Opin Rheumatol 2015;27(1):1–9.

26. Lalani TA, Kanne JP, Hatfield GA, et al. Imaging findings in systemic lupus erythematosus. Radiographics 2004;24(4):1069–86.

27. Sran S, Sran M, Patel N, et al. Lupus enteritis as an initial presentation of systemic lupus erythematosus. Case Rep Gastrointest Med 2014;2014:962735.

28. Ha HK, Lee SH, Rha SE, et al. Radiologic features of vasculitis involving the gastrointestinal tract. Radiographics 2000;20(3):779–94.

29. Fintelmann F, Levine MS, Rubesin SE. Jejunal diverticulosis: findings on CT in 28 patients. AJR Am J Roentgenol 2008;190(5):1286–90.

30. Stacey R, Green JT. Radiation-induced small bowel disease: latest developments and clinical guidance. Ther Adv Chronic Dis 2014;5(1):15–29.

31. Capps GW, Fulcher AS, Szucs RA, et al. Imaging features of radiation-induced changes in the abdomen. Radiographics 1997;17(6):1455–73.

32. Viswanathan C, Bhosale P, Ganeshan DM, et al. Imaging of complications of oncological therapy in the gastrointestinal system. Cancer Imaging 2012;12:163–72.

33. Lubner MG, Menias CO, Agrons M, et al. Imaging of abdominal and pelvic manifestations of graft-versus-host disease after hematopoietic stem cell transplant. AJR Am J Roentgenol 2017;209(1):33–45.

34. Chang ST, Menias CO, Lubner MG, et al. Molecular and clinical approach to intra-abdominal adverse effects of targeted cancer therapies. Radiographics 2017;37(5):1461–82.

Magnetic Resonance of Small Bowel Tumors

Gabriele Masselli, MD, PhD*, Marianna Guida, MD, Francesca Laghi, MD, Elisabetta Polettini, MD, Gianfranco Gualdi, MD

KEYWORDS

• Small bowel neoplasms • MR imaging • MR staging • MR enteroclysis • MR enterography

KEY POINTS

- Small bowel tumors are rare neoplasms, representing less than 5% of all gastrointestinal tract tumors.
- Intraluminal and extraluminal magnetic resonance (MR) findings, combined with contrast enhancement and functional information, allow accurate diagnoses and characterization of small bowel neoplasms.
- MR enteroclysis is an imaging modality that combines the advantages of enteroclysis and multiplanar MR and should be recommended for the initial investigation in suspected small bowel tumors.

INTRODUCTION

Although the small intestine encompasses more than 90% of the mucosal surface area of the gastrointestinal tract, small bowel neoplasms are rare, accounting for 3% to 6% of all gastrointestinal tract neoplasms.[1,2]

Patients with bowel tumors can be asymptomatic or may present vague symptoms such as abdominal pain, weight loss, or gastrointestinal bleeding.[2,3]

The diagnosis is complicated further by the nonspecific nature of these symptoms and commonly by a low index of clinical suspicion, which makes the detection of these neoplasms a challenge for physicians and radiologists.[3]

Inadequate radiologic examinations or incorrect interpretation of radiologic findings may cause further delays in diagnosing primary neoplasms of the small intestine.[4]

Either benign or malign tumors may cause complications such as intussusception, obstruction, or perforation.

Although conventional enteroclysis and capsule endoscopy are the most common procedures for visualizing mucosal abnormalities of the small bowel, they cannot evaluate the mural and extramural extent of small bowel neoplasms, with no possibility of complete staging of the tumor. Computed tomography (CT) and magnetic resonance (MR) are frequently used in suspicion of tumor of the small bowel.[5–7]

Common small bowel tumors typically are well evaluated with cross-sectional imaging modalities such as CT and MR, but accurate identification and differentiation can be challenging. Differentiating normal bowel from abnormal tumor depends on imaging modality and the particular technique.

Although endoscopic evaluation is typically more sensitive for the detection of intraluminal tumors that can be reached, CT and MR, as well as select nuclear medicine studies, remain superior for evaluating extraluminal neoplasms.

MR imaging offers numerous advantages with its excellent soft tissue contrast resolution, multiplanar imaging capability, and a lack of ionizing radiation. Furthermore, data acquisition can be repeated over time for functional evaluation of small bowel mobility, which is helpful for diagnosing low-grade stenosis and determining the level of obstruction.[8–10]

Disclosure: The authors have nothing to disclose.
Radiology Department, Umberto I Hospital Sapienza University, Viale del Policlinico 155, Rome 00161, Italy
* Corresponding author.
E-mail address: gabriele.masselli@uniroma1.it

Understanding the imaging characteristics of typical benign and malignant small bowel tumors is critical, because of overlapping features and associated secondary complications.

SMALL BOWEL TUMORS

The most common benign tumors are lipoma, adenoma, leiomyoma, hemangioma, and gastrointestinal stromal tumor (GIST; this also exists in a malignant form), whereas the most frequent malignant tumors are lymphoma, neuroendocrine tumor, metastatic disease, and primary small bowel adenocarcinoma.

The appearance of the lesions on MR imaging, combined with the contrast enhancement behavior and the characteristics of stenosis, can help to differentiate neoplasms of the small bowel (the main features are shown in **Table 1**).

BENIGN TUMORS
Adenoma

Adenoma is the most common benign tumor of the small bowel. Adenomas are generally small (<2 cm) but may grow large enough to lead to obstruction or intussusception. The risk of malignant transformation in small bowel adenomas increases when their size exceeds 1 cm.[2,11,12]

Adenoma may present with 3 possible patterns: a polypoid pedunculated mass on a stalk, a sessile mass (broad based and without a stalk), and a mural nodule within the mucosa.

It appears as an intraluminal homogeneous enhancing mass on gadolinium-enhanced fat-suppressed images, confined within the boundaries of intestinal lumen. Single shot fast spin echo (ssFSE) and Steady state GRE sequences show a rounded low-signal-intensity intraluminal mass, whereas MR fluoroscopy sequences show an intraluminal filling defect with mild narrowing of the lumen, which is not usually associated with proximal dilatation[11] (**Fig. 1**).

Leiomyoma

Small bowel leiomyomas are rare mesenchymal neoplasms with a predilection for the esophagus, although, in the small bowel, they are more frequently in the jejunum than in the ileum.[1]

Depending on their location, leiomyomas may protrude into the lumen or produce a mass effect on adjacent bowel. A small bowel leiomyoma appears as a homogeneous focal round mass with intense uniform enhancement.[13]

Leiomyoma shows benign features with uniform enhancement greater than that of adjacent bowel on postgadolinium images, without mesenteric involvement or metastases. On MR fluoroscopy, leiomyoma appears as a smooth, round, or semilunar mural defect that is demarcated by sharp angles to the intestinal wall.

Lipoma

Lipomas are mature adipose tissue proliferations arising in the submucosa of the bowel wall; the

---

Table 1
Magnetic resonance features of small bowel neoplasms

Histology	Common Site	T$_1$ Signal	T$_2$ Signal	Contrast Enhancement	MR Fluoroscopy
Adenoma	Jejunum	Low	High	Marked homogeneous	Intraluminal submucosa
Leiomyoma	Proximal ileum	Low	Low	Marked homogeneous	Intraluminal submucosal/extraluminal
Lipoma	Ileum	High	High; low at fat saturation	Absence	Intraluminal
Hemangioma	Jejunum	Low	High	Marked heterogeneous	Normal
GIST	Jejunum	Low	High heterogeneous	Marked heterogeneous	Extramural
Adenocarcinoma	Jejunum	Low	Low	Mild heterogeneous	Annular narrowing
Carcinoid	Distal ileum	Low	Low	Marked homogeneous	Intraluminal submucosal narrowing kinking
Lymphoma	Ileum	Low	Low	Mild heterogeneous	Stenosis or dilatation

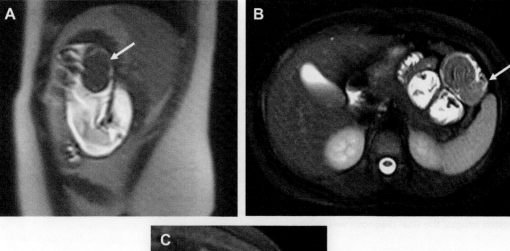

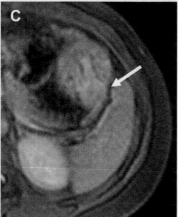

Fig. 1. MR imaging shows a jejunal adenoma on (*A, B*) T$_2$ ssFSE images, which appears as a rounded, polypoid, low-signal-intensity intraluminal mass (*arrow* in *A* and *B*) in the proximal jejunum (*arrow* in *C*) and causes (*B, C*) dilatation and intussusception.

ileum is the most frequent location. They usually grow intraluminally but occasionally extend outward in the mesenteric surface.[13]

Submucosal lipomas appear as sharply demarcated, sessile, small intraluminal lesions with high signal on T$_1$-weighted images and isointensity comparable with intra-abdominal fat on T$_2$-weighted images. On T$_1$-weighted and T$_2$-weighted fat-suppressed images these lesions show a loss of signal intensity. After gadolinium injection, lipomas show no enhancement (**Fig. 2**).

Hemangioma

Intestinal hemangiomas are usually submucosal tumors, most frequently located in the jejunum, and are sessile or pedunculate.

Hemangiomas show low signal intensity on T$_1$-weighted images and marked hyperintensity on T$_2$-weighted images; marked nodular enhancement is seen within the tumor in the arterial phase

and homogeneous enhancement in the delayed phase (**Fig. 3**).

Diffuse angiomatosis of the ileum appears as multiple nodules with low signal intensity on T$_1$-weighted images and marked hypersignal on T$_2$-weighted images; central nodular enhancement is seen within the tumor in the arterial phase with centrifugal enhancement on delayed phase.

BENIGN/MALIGNANT TUMORS
Gastrointestinal Stromal Tumor

GIST is the most common mesenchymal neoplasm of the gastrointestinal tract, including both benign and malignant varieties, and they are most commonly seen in patients more than 40 years of age.[14]

GISTs arise from interstitial cells of Cajal and almost always express a specific tyrosine kinase growth factor receptor known as c-KIT (cluster of differentiation [CD] 117), which differentiates them from true leiomyomas. Seventy percent of

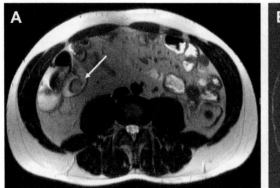 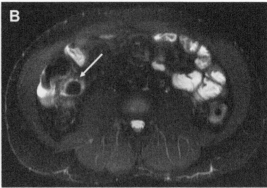

Fig. 2. MR imaging shows demarcated intraluminal lesion on terminal ileum (*arrow* in *A* and *B*) that appears iso-intense to intra-abdominal fat on (*A*) T_2-weighted images with loss of signal intensity on (*B*) T_2-weighted fat-suppressed images; the final diagnosis was lipoma.

GISTs are located in the stomach, 20% to 30% in the small bowel, and 7% in the anus or rectum.

Unlike adenocarcinomas, GISTs usually have an exophytic growth with involvement of the outer muscular layer of the bowel. Ulceration of the mucosa is seen in 50% of cases.[15,16]

On MR imaging, a GIST typically appears as an exophytic, sometimes bulky mass that can extend to several centimeters in size, displacing the adjacent bowel loops.

Following intravenous administration of contrast media, GISTs are typically enhancing masses with areas of low attenuation from hemorrhage, necrosis, or cyst formation.[17]

Unlike adenocarcinoma, GIST does not involve the bowel wall concentrically and consequently

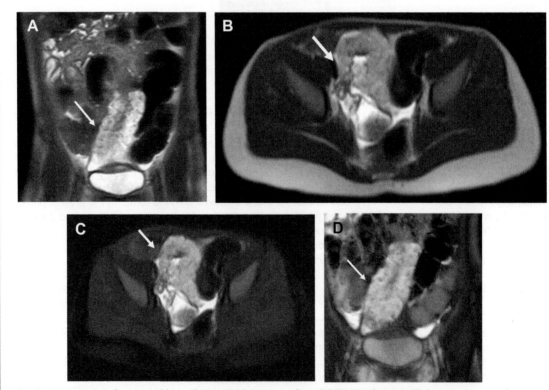

Fig. 3. MR imaging shows on (*A, B, C*) T_2 ssFSE images and on (*D*) T_2 steady state GRE sequences a submucosal tumor in the jejunum (*arrows* in *A–C*), marked hyperintense (*arrow* in *D*), which corresponds to a cavernous hemangioma.

bowel obstruction is rare, despite its large size. The intraluminal component accounts for a small proportion of tumors. The primary lesion is large and is the predominant finding. Mesenteric masses are usually well defined with a smooth surface without spiculation or indrawing of mesentery. Like lymphoma, GIST can also show aneurysmal dilatation of the bowel.[18]

Tumor diameter greater than 10 cm and local invasion are strong indicators of malignancy. However, even larger tumors tend to displace adjacent structures rather than invade. Malignant GISTs can present with metastases to the liver, omentum, and peritoneum (**Figs. 4** and **5**).[15,19,20]

MALIGNANT TUMORS
Adenocarcinoma

Primary small bowel carcinoma is rare, representing less than 2% of all gastrointestinal tumors, but is the most common primary small bowel malignancy. More than 50% of tumors are located in the duodenum, followed by the jejunum and then the ileum. Those arising from the jejunum are

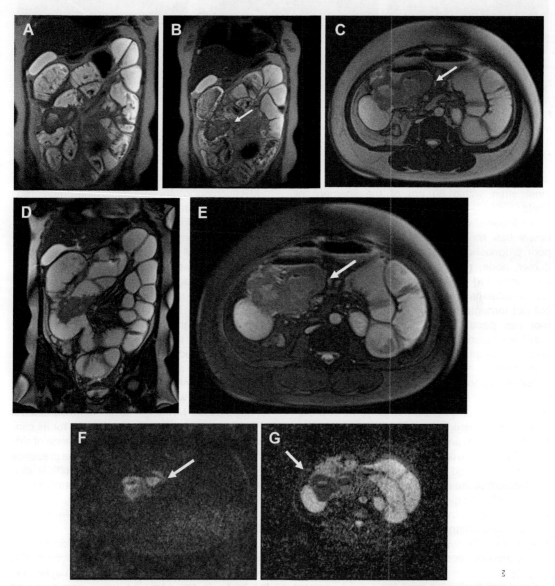

Fig. 4. MR imaging shows on (*arrow* in *B*) T$_2$ ssFSE images and on (*arrow* in *C* and *E*) T$_2$ steady state GRE a large lesion, with exophytic growth, located in the jejunum, without bowel obstruction. This GIST shows on (*arrow* in *F*) diffusion-weighted imaging (DWI) and on (*arrow* in *G*) apparent diffusion coefficient (ADC) sequences restricted diffusion caused by its high cellularity.

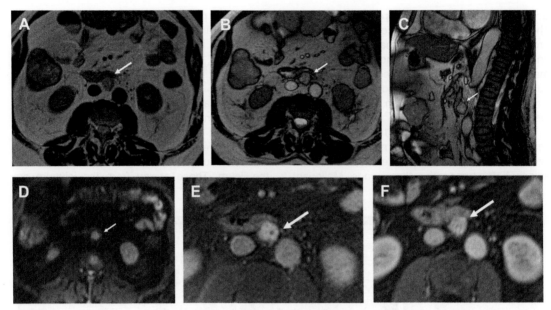

Fig. 5. MR imaging shows a GIST originating from the third duodenal portion, which appears as an exophytic mass slightly hyperintense on (*arrow* in *A*) T$_2$ turbo spin echo and on (*arrow* in *B* and *C*) T$_2$ steady state GRE sequences. It shows restricted diffusion (*arrow* in *D*) on DWI images and high contrast enhancement (*arrow* in *E* and *F*) after gadolinium injection.

most often within 30 cm of the ligament of Trietz.[2,21,22]

Small bowel primary adenocarcinoma of small bowel has an aggressive clinical nature with poor prognostic indicators including T3 disease (tumor, node, metastasis [TNM] staging: tumor has penetrated through the mucosa, submucosa, and muscularis propria and into the subserosa but not through the serosa) and T4 disease (tumor has penetrated through the serosa and may have invaded nearby tissues or organs), N1 and N2 lymph node metastasis, and distal metastasis.[23]

Adenocarcinomas may be polypoid, infiltrating, or stenosing. Duodenal adenocarcinomas are often more circumscribed, with polypoid or protuberant appearance, whereas jejunal or ileal lesions tend to be larger, annular, constricting tumors with circumferential involvement of the intestine wall. It is common to find fully parietal penetration and involvement of the serosal surface.[24,25]

On MR imaging, adenocarcinomas may appear as infiltrative lesions that cause luminal stenosis and obstruction with prestenotic dilatation, whereas polypoid intraluminal masses are less common; ulceration is a common feature (**Fig. 6**).

Focal wall thickening involving a short segment that shows hypointensity on T$_2$-weighted images and a heterogeneous moderate enhancement on gadolinium images is frequently seen.[26]

MR fluoroscopy shows luminal high-grade irregular stenosis with a fixed, unchanging appearance during the infusion of the intraluminal contrast.

Adenocarcinomas tend to infiltrate the entire bowel wall and extend into the surrounding mesenteric fat tissue, causing a local desmoplastic reaction. MR imaging is also able to stage liver metastases, lymph node involvement, and peritoneal carcinomatosis. The comparative characteristics favoring the diagnosis of primary adenocarcinoma include that it is a solitary lesion, it is most frequently located proximally, it involves short segments of bowel, and it infiltrates perivisceral fat.[11]

Extraluminal infiltration may present hyperintensity of the outer wall layers and fat on T$_2$-weighted fat-suppressed MR sequences. Adenocarcinoma of the ileum may mimic Crohn disease for its clinical and radiologic features but the absence of significant engorgement of the vasa and the presence of a single focal lesion rather than multiple skip areas of wall thickening may be useful criteria to suspect malignancy.[27]

Carcinoid

Carcinoid tumors are a type of neuroendocrine tumor (NET) that arises from the enterochromaffin cells and can affect virtually any organ system in the body. In the past, the terms carcinoid and neuroendocrine tumor were used interchangeably, but not all neuroendocrine cell tumors are carcinoids.[28]

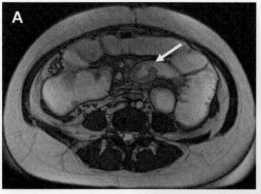
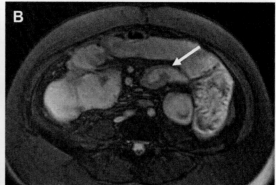
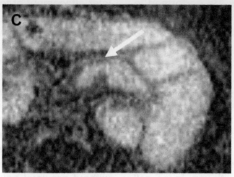

Fig. 6. MR imaging shows on (*A*) T$_2$ steady state GRE and on (*B*) T$_2$ steady state GRE fat sat images a focal wall thickening (*arrow* in *A* and *B*) involving a short segment of the jejunum. It presents restricted diffusion (*arrow* in *C*) on ADC images. Final biopsy identified a jejunal adenocarcinoma.

Carcinoid is the second most common malignancy, accounting for approximately 20% to 25% of all small bowel neoplasms, although its frequency has recently been reported to be increased up to 35%.[27]

Duodenal carcinoids are clinically and histopathologically distinct from jejunal and ileal NETs because they rarely arise from enterochromaffin cells.[29]

The ileum is the most common site of carcinoid tumors in the small bowel. The tumors arise from enterochromaffin cells and are equally distributed in men and women, with mean age of 65.4 years.[30]

Patients can be asymptomatic or present with abdominal pain, weight loss, melena, bowel obstruction, and ischemia.[31]

Bowel obstruction or abdominal pain could be caused by intussusceptions or mesenteric ischemia caused by local fibrosis of the adjacent mesentery.[32]

Metastases and secondary features such as desmoplasia and vascular involvement are often more easily visualized on MR imaging than the primary tumor, which tends to be small (1–2 cm) and difficult to find.[33]

On imaging, duodenal carcinoids can appear as intraluminal polyps and mural masses with early arterial enhancement and delayed washout, and present hypointensity on T$_1$-weighted images and heterogeneously hyperintensity on T$_2$-weighted images with heterogeneous enhancement. Tumors greater than 2 cm that infiltrate the muscularis propria and that show high mitotic activity are more prone to metastases.[32,34]

Jejunal and ileal carcinoid tumors cause focal, asymmetric bowel wall thickening and usually manifest as nodular wall thickening or a smooth submucosal mass. On unenhanced sequences, these lesions are isointense to muscle on T$_1$-weighted images and isointense or mildly hyperintense to muscle on T$_2$-weighted images. The primary lesions show contrast enhancement, especially on arterial phase.[3]

MR fluoroscopy shows solitary or multiple round, intramural, or intraluminal filling defects encroaching on the intestinal lumen; if a secondary mesenteric mass is present, it can manifest with stretching, rigidity, and fixation of ileal loops. Carcinoid neoplasm causes kinking of the bowel wall, with secondary narrowing of the lumen, rather than annular stenosis.[1,35]

The characteristic desmoplastic changes in the mesentery and retroperitoneum are caused by the secretion of serotonin and tryptophan and may present as an oval soft tissue mesenteric mass with radiating linear strands and thickened adjacent bowel loops with low signal on both T_1-weighted and T_2-weighted images, and may show negligible enhancement after contrast (**Fig. 7**).[13,26]

Combining the advantages of high soft tissue contrast together with superior alignment quality, fully integrated PET/MR imaging systems represent a promising alternative to PET/CT for patients with NET. A protocol containing T_2 HASTE, T_2 turbo spin echo, and diffusion-weighted imaging for nonenhanced PET/MR imaging with somatostatine receptors-specific radiotracers of the abdomen can be performed in a comparable time and with comparable effectiveness in lesion detection as a multiphase contrast-enhanced PET/CT.[36]

Lymphoma

Lymphoma represents the third most common neoplasm, accounting for 15% to 20% of all malignant small bowel tumors, with more than 60% arising from the ileum.[37–39]

Almost all the primary gastrointestinal lymphomas are of B-cell lineage, with very few T-cell lymphomas and classic Hodgkin lymphoma.[40]

The most important risk factors are immune suppression, celiac disease, and acquired immunodeficiency syndrome.

The terminal ileum is the most frequent site, owing to the increased amount of lymphoid tissue normally present relative to the duodenum and jejunum.

Intestinal lymphoma can assume different gross appearances: diffusely infiltrating lesions that often produce full-thickness mural thickening with effacement of overlying mucosal folds; polypoid lesions that protrude into the lumen; large, exophytic, and fungating masses that are prone to ulceration and fistula formation.[41]

The infiltrative form is characterized by circumferentially infiltrating lymphoma and involves a variable length of small bowel with thickening and later effacement of folds.

The polypoid pattern may cause bowel intussusceptions and shows solid nodules with homogeneous signal intensity developing as polypoid mass; the wall thickening is rarely associated. The aneurysmal pattern usually coexists with the infiltrative form and it can represent its evolution.[40]

In the setting of diffuse infiltrating lesions, the bowel wall appears dilated, possibly because of interference with the normal innervation and regulation of smooth muscle bowel wall contraction. The presence of a bowel wall mass and dilatation without proximal bowel obstruction is suggestive of lymphoma. Aneurysmal dilatation of the small bowel caused by loss of muscle tone of the intestinal wall is caused by lymphomatous invasion and destruction of the muscle layers and neural

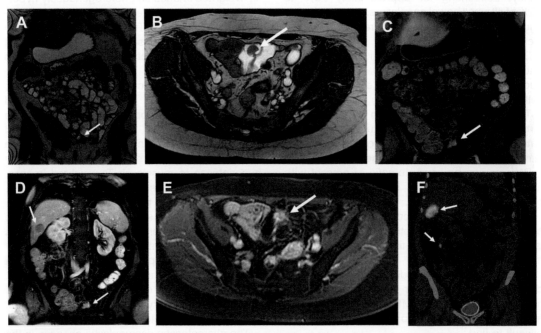

Fig. 7. (*A*) MR imaging T_2 steady state GRE coronal (*arrow*) and (*B*) axial (*arrow*) images show a small nodular lesion in an ileal loop in hypogastric region. After contrast injection (*arrows* in *C–E*), it presents high vascularization, with evidence of a liver metastasis (*arrow* in *D*) on segment VI. ^{18}F-FDOPA PET/CT (*arrows* in *F*) confirms the diagnosis of carcinoid tumor.

plexuses. The presence of diffuse splenomegaly and mesenteric and retroperitoneal lymphadenopathy supports the diagnosis.[3]

On MR fluoroscopic sequences, small bowel lymphoma appears as an infiltrative lesion with patency of bowel lumen or a nonstenotic bowel mass (**Figs. 8** and **9**).

Central ulceration has been described as a target lesion. The mesenteric form of small bowel lymphoma may present multiple small bowel masses, with displacement or compression of bowel loops or adjacent vessels. Coexisting lymphadenopathy encasing the mesenteric vasculature produces the classic sandwich sign.[42]

A large, aggressive, ulcerated adenocarcinoma can easily be mistaken for lymphoma; however, infiltration of mesenteric fat is more likely to be seen in adenocarcinoma. Moreover, lymph node metastases in lymphoma are usually more bulky than in adenocarcinoma.

Metastases

Metastases account for approximately 50% of all small bowel neoplasms and are the most probable tumors in patients with known neoplasms. Metastases develop through 4 major pathways: direct extension, intraperitoneal seeding, lymphatic spread, and hematogenous spread.[13]

Small bowel represents the main site of metastatic disease in the gastrointestinal tract. Although GISTs, adenocarcinoma, and carcinoid tumors often metastasize to the small intestine, the most frequent extra-abdominal causes of small intestine metastases are melanoma, lung, breast, and thyroid cancers.[43,44]

Metastatic lesions often lodge on the antimesenteric border of the small bowel. On gadolinium-enhanced fat-suppressed spoiled gradient-echo images, hypervascular metastases

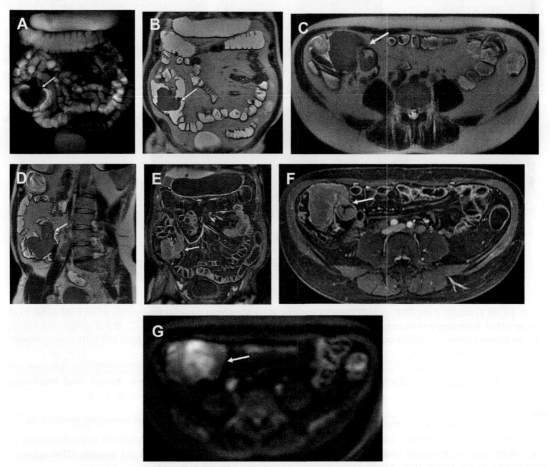

Fig. 8. MR imaging shows (*arrow* in A) a diffusely infiltrating lymphoma that originates from terminal ileum and involves the cecum. On (*B*) coronal, (*C*) axial, and (*D*) parasagittal T_2-weighted images, it appears as a circumferentially infiltrating mass without significant stenosis (*arrows* in B–D). After gadolinium injection, it shows (*arrows* in E and F) poor contrast enhancement. On DWI sequences, it presents (*arrow* in G) restricted diffusion for its high cellularity.

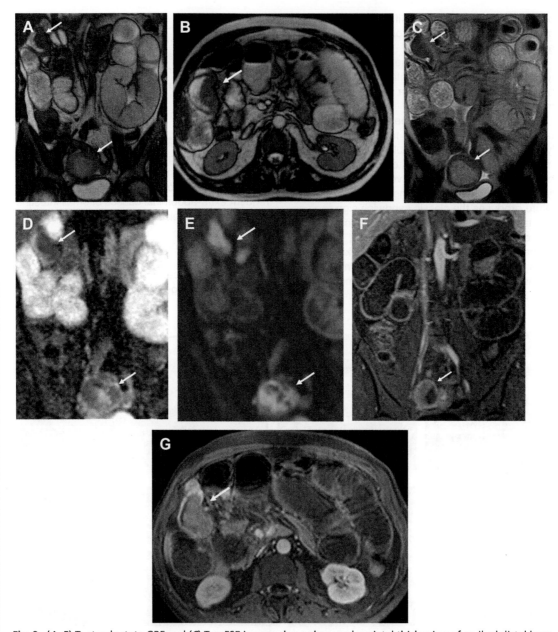

Fig. 9. (*A, B*) T$_2$ steady state GRE and (*C*) T$_2$ ssFSE images show abnormal parietal thickening of an ileal distal loop with another pathologic thickening in jejunal in right hypochondrium (*arrows* in *A–C*). These lymphoma localizations present restricted diffusion on (*arrows* in *D*) ADC and (*arrows* in *E*) DWI and mild contrast enhancement (*arrows* in *F* and *G*) after gadolinium.

are moderately high in signal intensity, in contrast with the low signal intensity of intra-abdominal fat.[45]

Metastatic involvement of the small bowel usually appears as a smooth, round, or polypoid mass that can be ulcerated and may cause intussusception or occlusion (**Fig. 10**).[46]

Metastases in the small bowel can also occur as extramural nodules following intraperitoneal seeding, especially from primary mucinous tumors, and may cause an increase in bowel wall thickness with infiltration of the mesenteric fat.[47]

Leiomyosarcoma
Leiomyosarcomas arise from the smooth muscle of the wall or from small blood vessels. The appearance can be similar to that of leiomyomas except for the size, which usually exceeds 5 cm. Leiomyosarcoma grows slowly, predominantly extraluminally and eccentrically, and appears as a large

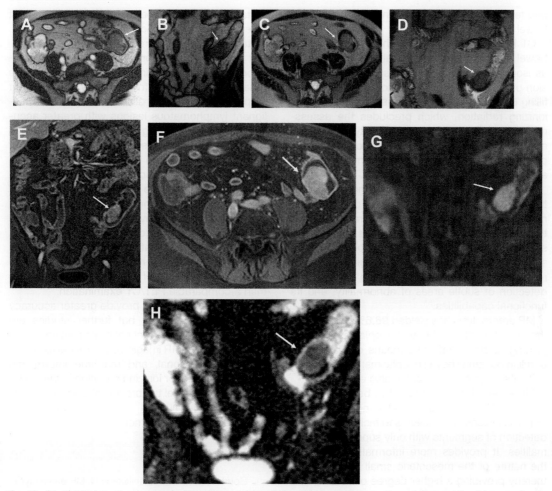

Fig. 10. (*A, B*) MR imaging T$_2$ steady state GRE and (*C, D*) T$_2$ ssFSE images show, in a patient with a history of melanoma, a metastatic jejunal localization (*arrows in A–D*) in the left iliac fossa. It presents strong contrast enhancement on dynamic phases (*arrows in E and F*) and restricted diffusion on (*arrow in G*) DWI and (*arrow in H*) ADC images.

heterogeneous mass with central necrosis and hemorrhage. MR fluoroscopy shows a large extrinsic mass, displacing or distorting adjacent loops.[11]

Compared with their benign counterparts leiomyomas, MR criteria favoring malignancy include a large size (6 cm) and areas of necrosis or heterogeneous tissue intensity.

ROLE OF MAGNETIC RESONANCE IMAGING COMPARED WITH OTHER MODALITIES

Although conventional enteroclysis and capsule endoscopy represent the most common procedures for visualizing mucosal abnormalities of the small bowel, their use may be limited by clinical conditions, with no possibility of evaluating the mural and extramural extent of these neoplasms.[48]

The use of capsule endoscopy to evaluate small bowel tumors, particularly submucosal forms, has several limitations, such as the difficulty in identifying the abnormality and tumor type based on the capsule endoscopic appearance of the lesions. Capsule endoscopy may fail to detect neoplastic disease in as many as 18.9% of cases, and the capsule retention is seen in 10% to 25% of cases of small bowel tumor.[49–52]

Barium studies have low accuracy in detecting small bowel neoplasms because of their segmental distension of bowel loop (with consequently suboptimal distension) and the difficulty in evaluating overlapping intestinal loops.

MR and CT techniques optimized for small bowel imaging are useful tools in the evaluation of small bowel disorders. Several studies have shown the advantages of these techniques compared with traditional barium fluoroscopic examinations because of improvements in spatial and temporal resolution combined with improved bowel distending agents.

CT is a useful modality in the investigation of bowel masses but has several limitations, such as isoattenuating lesions and suboptimal distension of the lumen. It cannot monitor small bowel filling in real time without exposing the patient to ionizing radiation, which precludes the assessment of small bowel peristaltic activity. In addition, an intermittent spasm or peristaltic contraction during the examination can also be misdiagnosed as a small bowel neoplasm on the CT study.[53,54]

MR enterography seems to be more accurate than CT enterography in the detection of neoplastic diseases. It is a well-tolerated imaging technique that accurately depicts mesenteric small bowel tumors because of the better soft tissue contrast afforded by MR imaging, which is required for tissue characterization and for the detection of subtle areas of abnormality, and its functional capabilities.[55]

MR enteroclysis has yielded 96.6% accuracy in the detection of small bowel neoplasms, thereby proving to be an effective means of diagnosing or ruling out small bowel neoplasms; interobserver MR enteroclysis agreement is also excellent.[35]

MR enteroclysis has proved to be more sensitive than CT enteroclysis in detecting small bowel mucosal lesions, and it seems to facilitate superior detection of segments with only superficial abnormalities. It provides more information regarding the nature of the mesenteric small bowel tumor, thereby providing a higher degree of small bowel tumor characterization.[56,57]

[18]F-radiolabeled amino acids, such as 18F-FLUORO-DOPA (^{18}F-FDOPA), have been successfully proposed as PET/CT imaging agents for small bowel neuroendocrine tumors for the avid demand of amine precursors of neuroendocrine cells. The high uptake of ^{18}F-FDOPA in NETs is the result of the increased synthesis, storage, and secretion of biogenic amines, such as dopamine and serotonin.[58]

The addition of [18]F- FDOPA PET/CT to standard radiologic imaging (CT, MR imaging) during the preoperative work-up of patients with small bowel NETs significantly increases the detection rate of primary tumor and liver metastasis.[59]

Fluorodeoxyglucose (FDG) PET is an important tool in oncological patient management, especially for disease staging, restaging, and monitoring response to treatment. FDG-PET/CT is useful in the initial diagnosis, disease staging, and evaluating response to treatment of small bowel adenocarcinoma. It allows the detection and characterization of local and distant lymph node involvement and unsuspected local and distant metastases. It can be used in posttreatment (chemotherapy or surgical) response assessment, restaging, and/or recurrence.[60]

It is also accurate for baseline staging of lymphoma and for determining the most appropriate initial treatment. Used for evaluation of treatment response, PET/CT can depict residual viable malignant lymphomatous lesions with greater accuracy than other imaging techniques. The findings thereby influence decisions about the need for additional or alternative treatment.[60]

FDG-PET/CT can also play a role in the detection and in the disease response assessment of GIST and small bowel metastases (eg, melanoma).

PET/MR enterography is technically feasible as an imaging technique to assess bowel lesions in malignant and inflammatory disease. The radiation exposure to patients having this procedure is reduced by at least half and is up to 4 times less than a comparable PET/CT examination.

PET/MR imaging may provide greater accuracy in neoplastic detection but further studies are needed to define its practical clinical value.[61,62]

In conclusion, MR imaging can provide exquisite anatomic, functional, and real-time information without the need for ionizing radiation in the evaluation of small bowel tumors and should be recommended for evaluating patients suspected of having a small bowel tumor.

REFERENCES

1. Gourtsoyiannis N, Papanikolaou N. MR enteroclysis. In: Gore R, Levine M, editors. Textbook of gastrointestinal radiology. 3rd edition. Philadelphia (PA): Saunders Elsevier; 2008. p. 765–74.

2. Williams EA, Bowman AW. Multimodality imaging of small bowel neoplasms. Abdom Radiol (NY) 2019; 44(6):2089–103.

3. Masselli G, Casciani E, Polettini E, et al. Magnetic resonance imaging of small bowel neoplasms. Cancer Imaging 2013;13:92–9.

4. Negaard A, Paulsen V, Sandvik L, et al. A prospective randomized comparison between two MRI studies of the small-bowel in Crohn's disease, the oral contrast method and MR enteroclysis. Eur Radiol 2007;17:2294–301.

5. Masselli G, Casciani E, Polettini E, et al. Comparison of MR-enteroclysis with MR enterography and conventional enteroclysis in patients with Crohn's disease. Eur Radiol 2008;18:438–47.

6. Masselli G, Picarelli A, Di Tola M, et al. Celiac disease: Evaluation with dynamic contrast-enhanced MR imaging. Radiology 2010;256(3):783–90.

7. Masselli G, Picarelli A, Gualdi G. Celiac disease: MR enterography and contrast enhanced MRI. Abdom Imaging 2010;35(4):399–406.

8. Masselli G, Polettini E, Casciani E, et al. Small-bowel neoplasm: prospective evaluation of MR enteroclysis. Radiology 2009;251:743–50.

9. Fidler JL, Guimaraes L, Einstein DM. MR imaging of the small bowel. Radiographics 2009;29(6): 1811–25.

10. Amzallag-Bellenger E, Soyer P, Barbe C, et al. Diffusion-weighted imaging for the detection of mesenteric small bowel tumours with Magnetic Resonance-enterography. Eur Radiol 2014;24(11): 2916–26.

11. Masselli G, Colaiacomo MC, Marcelli G, et al. MRI of the small-bowel: how to differentiate primary neoplasms and mimickers. Br J Radiol 2012;85:824–37.

12. De Latour RA, Kilaru SM, Gross SA. Management of small bowel polyps: a literature review. Best Pract Res Clin Gastroenterol 2017;31(4):401–8.

13. Lappas JC, Maglinte DD, Sandrasegaran K. Benign tumors of the small bowel. In: Gore R, Levine M, editors. Textbook of gastrointestinal radiology. 3rd edition. Philadelphia (PA): Saunders Elsevier; 2008. p. 845–51.

14. Rabin I, Chikman B, Lavy R, et al. Gastrointestinal stromal tumors: a 19 year experience. Isr Med Assoc J 2009;11(2):98–102.

15. Levy AD, Remotti HE, Thompson WM, et al. Gastrointestinal stromal tumors: radiologic features with pathologic correlation. Radiographics 2003;23(2): 283–304.

16. Ba-Ssalamah A, Prokop M, Uffmann M, et al. Dedicated multidetector CT of the stomach: spectrum of diseases. Radiographics 2003;23(3):625–44.

17. Shojaku H, Futatsuya R, Seto H, et al. Malignant gastrointestinal stromal tumor of the small intestine: radiologic-pathologic correlation. Radiat Med 1997;15:189–92.

18. Sandrasegaran K, Rajesh A, Rydberg J, et al. Gastrointestinal stromal tumors: clinical, radiologic, and pathologic features. AJR Am J Roentgenol 2005;184(3):803–11.

19. Suster S. Gastrointestinal stromal tumors. Semin Diagn Pathol 2009;13(4):297–313.

20. Crosby JA, Catton CN, Davis A, et al. Malignant gastrointestinal stromal tumors of the small intestine: A review of 50 cases from a prospective database. Ann Surg Oncol 2001;8(1):50–9.

21. McLaughlin PD, Maher MM. Primary malignant diseases of the small intestine. Am J Roentgenol 2013;201(1):W9–14.

22. Gore RM, Mehta UK, Berlin JW, et al. Diagnosis and staging of small bowel tumours. Cancer imaging 2006;6(1):209–12.

23. Chang H-K, Yu E, Kim J, et al. Adenocarcinoma of the small intestine: a multi-institutional study of 197 surgically resected cases. Hum Pathol 2010;41: 1087–96.

24. Ouriel K, Adams JT. Adenocarcinoma of the small intestine. Am J Surg 1984;147:66–71.

25. Zeh H III. Cancer of the small intestine. In: DeVita VT Jr, Hellman S, Rosenberg SA, editors. Cancer: principles and practice of oncology. 7th edition. Philadelphia (PA): Lippincott Williams & Wilkins; 2005. p. 1035–48.

26. Semelka RC, John G, Kelekis NL, et al. Small bowel neoplastic disease: demonstration by MRI. J Magn Reson Imaging 1996;6:855–60.

27. Anzidei M, Napoli A, Zini C, et al. Malignant tumours of the small intestine: a review of histopathology, multidetector CT and MRI aspects. Br J Radiol 2011;84(1004):677–90.

28. Klöppel G. Classification and pathology of gastroentero-pancreatic neuroendocrine neoplasms. Endocr Relat Cancer 2011;18(suppl 1): S1–16.

29. Levy AD, Sobin LH. Gastrointestinal carcinoids: imaging features with clinicopathologic comparison. Radiographics 2007;27(1):237–57.

30. Modlin IM, Lye KD, Kidd M. A 5-decade analysis of 13,715 carcinoid tumors. Cancer 2003;97(4): 934–59.

31. Elsayes KM, Menias CO, Bowerson M, et al. Imaging of carcinoid tumors: spectrum of findings with pathologic and clinical correlation. J Comput Assist Tomogr 2011;35(1):72–80.

32. Baxi AJ, Chintapalli K, Katkar A, et al. Multimodality imaging findings in carcinoid tumors: a head-to-toe spectrum. Radiographics 2017;37(2):516–36.

33. Woodbridge LR, Murtagh BM, Yu DF, et al. Midgut neuroendocrine tumors: imaging assessment for surgical resection. Radiographics 2014;34(2): 413–26.

34. Levy AD, Taylor LD, Abbott RM, et al. Duodenal carcinoids: imaging features with clinical-pathologic comparison. Radiology 2005;237(3):967–72.

35. Van Weyenberg SJ, Meijerink MR, Jacobs MA, et al. MR Enteroclysis in the diagnosis of small-bowel neoplasms. Radiology 2010;254:765–73.

36. Seith F, Schraml C, Reischl G, et al. Fast non enhanced abdominal examination protocols in PET/MRI for patients with neuroendocrine tumors (NET): comparison to multiphase contrast-enhanced PET/CT. Radiol Med 2018;123(11): 860–70.

37. Cheung DY, Choi M. Current advance in small bowel tumors. Clin Endosc 2011;44(1):13–21.

38. Bäck H, Gustavsson B, Ridell B, et al. Primary gastrointestinal lymphoma incidence, clinical presentation, and surgical approach. J Surg Oncol 1986;33(4):234–8.

39. Ghimire P, Wu GY, Zhu L. Primary gastrointestinal lymphoma. World J Gastroenterol 2011;17(6): 697–707.

40. Pezzella M, Brogna B, Romano A, et al. Detecting a rare composite small bowel lymphoma by Magnetic Resonance Imaging coincidentally: a case report with radiological, surgical and histopathological features. Int J Surg Case Rep 2018;46:50–5.

41. Masselli G, Gualdi G. Evaluation of small bowel tumors: MR enteroclysis. Abdom Imaging 2010; 35(1):23–30.

42. Lo Re G, Federica V, Midiri F, et al. Radiological features of gastrointestinal lymphoma. Gastroenterol Res Pract 2016;2016:2498143.

43. Lens M, Bataille V, Krivokapic Z. Melanoma of the small intestine. Lancet Oncol 2009;10:516–21.

44. Phillips DL, Benner KG, Keeffe EB, et al. Isolated metastasis to small bowel from anaplastic thyroid carcinoma. With a review of extra-abdominal malignancies that spread to the bowel. J Clin Gastroenterol 1987;9:563–7.

45. Masselli G, Brizi MG, Restaino G, et al. MR enteroclysis in solitary ileal metastasis from renal cell carcinoma. AJR Am J Roentgenol 2004;182:828–9.

46. Sailer J, Zacherl J, Schima W. MDCT of small bowel tumours. Cancer Imaging 2007;7:224–33.

47. Sheth S, Horton KM, Garland MR, et al. Mesenteric neoplasms: CT appearances of primary and secondary tumors and differential diagnosis. Radiographics 2003;23:457–73.

48. Fork FT, Aabakken L. Capsule enteroscopy and radiology of the small intestine. Eur Radiol 2007; 17:3103–11.

49. Postgate A, Despott E, Burling D, et al. Significant small-bowel lesions detected by alternative diagnostic modalities after negative capsule endoscopy. Gastrointest Endosc 2008;68(6):1209–14.

50. Baichi MM, Arifuddin RM, Mantry PS. Small-bowel masses found and missed on capsule endoscopy for obscure bleeding. Scand J Gastroenterol 2007; 42(9):1127–32.

51. Pennazio M, Rondonotti E, de Franchis R. Capsule endoscopy in neoplastic diseases. World J Gastroenterol 2008;14(34):5245–53.

52. Estèvez E, Gonzàlez-Conde B, Vàzquez-Iglesias JL, et al. Incidence of tumoral pathology according to study using capsule endoscopy for patients with obscure gastrointestinal bleeding. Surg Endosc 2007;21(10):1776–80.

53. Masselli G, Gualdi G. CT and MR enterography in evaluating small bowel diseases: when to use which modality? Abdom Imaging 2013;38:249–59.

54. Maglinte DD, Sandrasegaran K, Lappas JC, et al. CT enteroclysis. Radiology 2007;245(3):661–71.

55. Masselli G, Di Tola M, Casciani E, et al. Diagnosis of small-bowel diseases: prospective comparison of multidetector row CT enterography with MR enterography. Radiology 2016;279(2):420–31.

56. Torkzad MR, Masselli G, Halligan S, et al. Indications and selection of MR enterography vs. MR enteroclysis with emphasis on patients who need small bowel MRI and general anaesthesia: results of a survey. Insights Imaging 2015;6(3):339–46.

57. Masselli G, Polettini E, Laghi F, et al. Noninflammatory conditions of the small bowel. Magn Reson Imaging Clin N Am 2014;22(1):51–65.

58. Fiebrich HB, de Jong JR, Kema IP, et al. Total (18) F-dopa PET tumour uptake reflects metabolic endocrine tumour activity in patients with a carcinoid tumour. Eur J Nucl Med Mol Imaging 2011;38: 1854–61.

59. Addeo P, Poncet G, Goichot B, et al. The added diagnostic value of 18F-Fluorodihydroxyphenylalanine PET/CT in the preoperative work-up of small bowel neuroendocrine tumors. J Gastrointest Surg 2018;22(4):722–30.

60. Cronin CG, Scott J, Kambadakone A, et al. Utility of positron emission tomography/CT in the evaluation of small bowel pathology. Br J Radiol 2012;85: 1211–21.

61. Beiderwellen K, Kinner S, Gomez B, et al. Hybrid imaging of the bowel using PET/MR enterography: Feasibility and first results. Eur J Radiol 2016; 85(2):414–21.

62. Masselli G, Gualdi G. MR imaging of the small bowel. Radiology 2012;264(2):333–48.

Magnetic Resonance Enema in Rectosigmoid Endometriosis

Ennio Biscaldi, MD[a],*, Fabio Barra, MD[b,c], Simone Ferrero, MD, PhD[b,c]

KEYWORDS

- Diagnosis • Endometriosis • MR imaging • Rectosigmoid endometriosis
- Rectosigmoid opacification

KEY POINTS

- Several studies showed the accuracy of MR-enema (MR-e) in the diagnosis of rectosigmoid endometriosis.
- During MR imaging, rectosigmoid opacification with ultrasound gel helps to delineate the intestinal wall, distinguishing it from the surrounding structures, and to identify intestinal endometriotic lesions.
- Despite intestinal distention and opacification, MR-e does not allow to distinguish the various layers of the intestinal wall in the normal colon (serosa, muscularis propria and mucosa).

INTRODUCTION

Endometriosis is a gynecologic condition characterized by the presence of endometriotic glands and stroma outside the uterine cavity. It affects at least 3.6% of reproductive age women[1] and it usually causes pain (dysmenorrhea, deep dyspareunia, nonmenstrual pelvic pain, dyschezia), infertility, and other symptoms, depending on the location of the lesions, such as urinary complaints in patients with bladder endometriosis and intestinal complaints in patients with bowel endometriosis. Endometriosis is usually classified in ovarian endometriosis, superficial endometriosis, and deep infiltrating endometriosis (DE). Ovarian endometriosis includes superficial ovarian implants and ovarian endometriotic cysts. Superficial endometriosis (also known as peritoneal endometriosis) is characterized by peritoneal infiltration of less than 5 mm depth. DE is the most severe form of the disease and is histologically defined as endometriosis infiltrating the retroperitoneum or the wall of pelvic organs by at least 5 mm.[2] DE may affect various pelvic organs and spaces including the posterior border of the cervix and isthmus of the uterus, uterosacral ligaments, paracervix, rectosigmoid, pouch of Douglas, bladder, vagina, and pelvic peritoneum.

Intestinal endometriosis is the most challenging form of endometriosis for the gynecologist. It occurs in 4% to 37% of women with DE.[3] The rectosigmoid colon is the most frequent location (about 85% of the cases), followed by the ileum, appendix, and cecum. The nonsurgical diagnosis of rectosigmoid endometriosis is necessary to offer the best treatment planning for the patients. Hormonal therapies have been shown to be effective in improving not only pain but also intestinal symptoms of patients with rectosigmoid

Disclosure: The authors have nothing to disclose.

[a] Department of Radiology, Galliera Hospital, via Mura delle Cappuccine 14, Genova 16128, Italy; [b] Academic Unit of Obstetrics and Gynaecology, IRCCS Ospedale Policlinico San Martino, Largo R. Benzi 10, 16132 Genoa, Italy; [c] Department of Neurosciences, Rehabilitation, Ophthalmology, Genetics, Maternal and Child Health (DiNOGMI), University of Genoa, Largo Paolo Daneo, 3, Genova 16132, Italy
* Corresponding author.
E-mail address: ennio.biscaldi@gmail.com

endometriosis.[4–7] Surgery is required in patients with subocclusive symptoms, in those with contra-indications to hormonal therapies or refusing these treatments, in those with symptoms persisting despite the use of hormonal therapies, and in those desiring to get pregnant, because all the available treatments are contraceptive or do not allow to conceive.[8] At laparoscopy, rectosigmoid endometriosis can be treated by nodulectomy, full-thickness disc resection, and segmental bowel resection. In patients undergoing surgery, it is important not only to establish the presence of rectosigmoid endometriosis but also to define the characteristics of the endometriotic nodules, such as the longitudinal diameter of the largest one, the depth of infiltration in the intestinal wall, the distance between the more caudal nodule and the anal verge, the presence of multifocal disease (presence of multiple lesions affecting the same segment), and the infiltration of adjacent organs.

OVERVIEW OF THE DIAGNOSIS OF RECTOSIGMOID ENDOMETRIOSIS

The presence of rectosigmoid endometriosis should be suspected when the typical endometriosis-related pain symptoms are associated with intestinal complains, such as abdominal bloating, intestinal cramping, painful bowel movements, constipation, and diarrhea (which often worsen during the menstrual cycle), and passage of mucus and rectal bleeding during the menstrual cycle.[3] These intestinal symptoms are very common, and, in particular, they are similar to those of irritable bowel syndrome.[9,10] The clinical examination (digital vaginal and rectal examination) may allow to detect a thickening or a nodule in the posterior vaginal fornix and rectum, which are suggestive of DE.[11,12] However, the physical examination does not allow a definitive diagnosis and it cannot detect endometriotic nodules located above the rectum. Therefore, imaging techniques are required for the diagnosis of rectosigmoid endometriosis.

Abdominal ultrasound has no role in the diagnosis of rectosigmoid endometriosis; however, it can be useful to exclude hydronephrosis caused by ureteral stenosis owing to endometriosis.[13] Several studies showed the accuracy of transrectal ultrasonography in the diagnosis of rectosigmoid endometriosis[14,15] but this examination is rarely used because of the discomfort caused by the procedure. Transvaginal ultrasonography (TVS) is currently the first-line investigation for the diagnosis of rectosigmoid endometriosis.[16]

A recent systematic review and metanalysis including 10 studies (2639 patients) showed that TVS has a sensibility of 91% and a specificity of 97% in diagnosing rectosigmoid endometriosis.[17] TVS has the advantage of being performed by gynecologists, which tend to have an expertise in treating patients with endometriosis, it is cheap and does not require bowel preparation.[18] However, TVS cannot detect nodules located proximally to the sigmoid because they are beyond the scope of this investigation. Furthermore, the diagnostic performance of TVS depends on the experience of the ultrasonographer. Improvement in the diagnostic accuracy of TVS may be obtained by introducing saline solution or gel in the vagina and/or rectum ("enhanced" or "modified" TVS),[19] as their distention may enhance the visualization of DE nodules.[20–24]

Endoscopic ultrasonography has been widely used to diagnose rectosigmoid endometriosis. This examination is particularly precise in estimating depth of infiltration of endometriosis in the intestinal wall, size and location of the nodules, and distance between the nodule and the anal verge.[25–29] Endoscopic ultrasonography and MR imaging have similar diagnostic performance in diagnosing rectosigmoid endometriosis[29]; however, the first is more precise than MR imaging in identifying the infiltration of the submucosa and mucosa.[30]

Double contrast barium enema (DCBE) has been widely used for the diagnosis of rectosigmoid endometriosis. This examination is easy to be performed and cheap,[31–35] but its use in the diagnosis of bowel endometriosis has some limitations: conventional radiology requires administration of ionizing radiation to women of reproductive age; DCBE requires an experienced radiologist, mainly in patients with suspicion of intestinal endometriosis; DCBE does not allow estimation of the depth of infiltration of endometriosis in the intestinal wall or the differentiation of bowel endometriosis from other intestinal pathologies, and, lastly, it does not identify the infiltration of adjacent organs.

Multidetector computerized tomography enema (MDCT-e) has a sensitivity of 98.7% and a specificity of 100% in diagnosing rectosigmoid endometriosis.[36] This examination has the advantage of identifying small endometriotic lesions located on the serosal surface, it may identify nodules located on the cecum and last ileal loops, and it precisely estimates the degree of infiltration of endometriosis in the intestinal wall.[37] Currently, new systems of dose control assist the radiologist in optimizing and decreasing the administered radiographic dose; for this reason, ionizing radiation is a minor limitation of MDCT when used to examine women of childbearing age.

However, the disadvantage of using iodinated contrast medium and exposing patients to radiation are 2 shortcomings of CT underlined many times in the literature. Furthermore, a recent study showed that MDCT-e and magnetic resonance enema (MR-e) have similar diagnostic performance in identifying rectosigmoid endometriosis.[38]

Virtual colonoscopy (CTC) has recently been used for the diagnosis of rectosigmoid endometriosis.[39–45] However, it not only requires bowel preparation, and the use of iodinated contrast medium during CTC is still controversial. A recent study showed that CTC and TVS have similar diagnostic performance in diagnosing rectosigmoid endometriosis; however, CTC is more panoramic and more precise in estimating the distance between the endometriotic nodules and the anal verge[45]; this parameter is particularly relevant for surgeons because patients with low rectal nodules tend to have an increased risk of ileostomy or colostomy at the time of surgery.

MR IMAGING IN THE DIAGNOSIS OF RECTOSIGMOID ENDOMETRIOSIS

MR imaging has long been considered the first-line investigation of the diagnosis of DE, including rectosigmoid endometriosis.[46] MR imaging should be performed on a 1 to 1.5 T magnet using at least an 8-channel pelvic phased array coil. The standard examination protocol includes the following sequences: T2-weighted fast relaxation fast spin echo (T2W FrFSE) axial images, T2W FrFSE fat sat coronal images, FIESTA (or similar) sequence in coronal plane, T2W FrSE sagittal images, T2W FrFSE fat sat sagittal images, and diffusion-weighted echo planar imaging (b = 1000, 1500) axial images. T1-weighted images are acquired using fat-suppression even after contrast enhancement (gadobutrol at a dosage of 0.2 mmol/kg body weight). This sequence allows differentiating between hemorrhagic and fatty content of adnexal cysts.[47] It is important to use an adequate field of view and a slice thickness of about 3 to 4 mm, particularly in case of nodules with main diameter of approximately 10 mm.

DIFFUSION-WEIGHTED IMAGING

Diffusion-weighted imaging (DWI) is now clinically accepted to detect and characterize focal lesions, to differentiate between malignant and benign lesions, and to monitor treatment response.[48]

However, the usefulness of DWI for differentiating benign from malignant ovarian cystic lesions is controversial, because teratomas and endometriomas tend also to have restricted diffusion.[49,50] Apparent diffusion coefficient (ADC) values has been used to identify endometriomas from hemorrhagic cysts, and these values may represent an additional diagnostic tool to differentiate them. However, as there was some overlap between the ADC values of endometriomas and hemorrhagic cysts, such diagnosis should be based on a combination of clinical history and conventional MR imaging with DWI findings, rather than based on DWI alone. To the best of our knowledge, there is no attempt of DWI clinical use in diagnosing rectosigmoid endometriosis; in our experience these sequences have no relevant role in the diagnosis of DE.

Concerning the use of paramagnetic contrast medium injection, whereas some authors obtain images before and after contrast,[51] other authors do not use contrast-enhanced imaging owing to the lack of a definite consensus on its usefulness. In fact, an accurate preoperative assessment of endometriosis extension, including deep implants and adhesions, has been demonstrated even without the use of gadolinium contrast medium.[52]

Rectosigmoid endometriosis usually contains extensive fibrosis and smooth muscle cells, with little or no endometriotic tissue[3] (Fig. 1). Therefore, DE usually has very similar signal intensity to that of the surrounding fibromuscular structures. Rectosigmoid endometriotic nodules appear as solid nodular thickening in the rectosigmoid wall; the lesion usually joins the

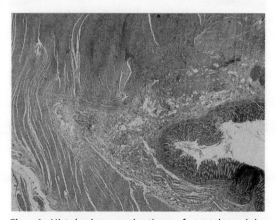

Fig. 1. Histologic examination of rectal nodule, showing multiple foci of endometriosis located in muscularis mucosa and submucosa with mild disarray of muscular fibers and perilesional fibrosis (hematoxylin and eosin staining).

intestinal wall at an obtuse angle and may have a stellar outline. The endometriotic nodule has a signal similar to that of the muscles in T1- and T2-weighted images. Its penetration in the intestinal wall with the subsequent disappearance of the fatty plan between the intestine and the nodule is the main parameter to diagnose infiltration of the muscularis propria. Mucosal involvement is rare; it may appear as a bulging transmural mass. Endometriotic foci appear sometime as spots of high signal intensity on T2- and T1-weighted images[47,53] (**Figs. 2** and **3**).

The radiological report should describe number and location of the nodules, degree of infiltration of endometriosis in the intestinal wall, maximum diameter of the nodules, distance between the lower border of the endometriotic nodule and the anal verge, and the presence of infiltration of adjacent organs (such as the vagina).

In 2004, a historical study by Bazot and colleagues[46] including 195 patients demonstrated that MR imaging with gadolinium contrast-enhanced sequences has high accuracy in diagnosing DE. In this study, MR imaging had an accuracy of 94.9% for diagnosing rectosigmoid involvement, a sensitivity of 88%, a specificity of 97.8%, a positive predictive value (PPV) of 95%, and a negative predictive value (NPV) of 95%. A recent systematic review and metanalysis including 6 studies (424 patients, of whom

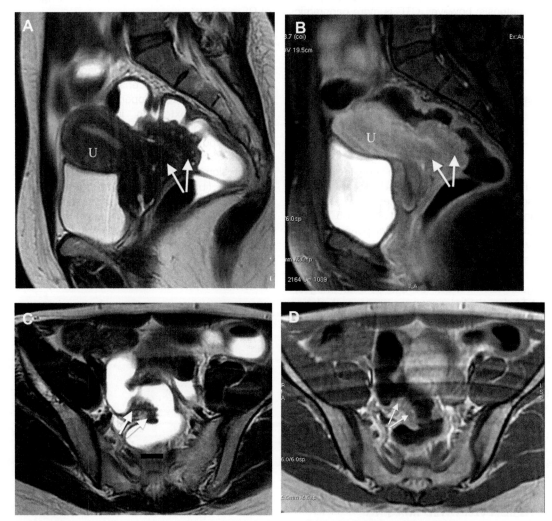

Fig. 2. MR-e: 24-year-old woman. (*A*) Sagittal fast echo spin (FSE) T2-weighted (T2W) sequence: endometriotic nodule infiltrating the low rectum (*arrows*). (*B*) FSE T1W fat sat sequence after paramagnetic contrast medium injection: poor enhancement of the lesion (*arrows*), very similar to the enhancement of the uterus (U). (*C*) Axial T2W sequence: the endometriotic nodule infiltrating the rectum is evident (*arrows*). (*D*) Axial image FSE T1W sequence: after contrast medium injection, the endometriotic nodule is still visible (*arrows*).

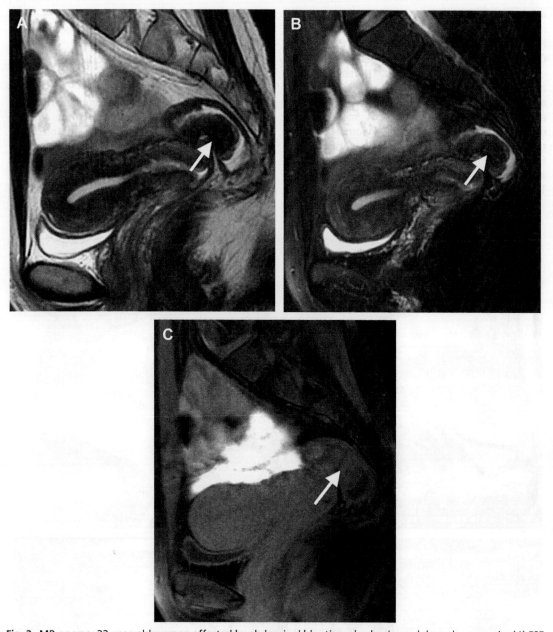

Fig. 3. MR-enema: 32-year-old woman affected by abdominal bloating, dyschezia, and deep dyspareunia. (*A*) FSE T2W sequence: the arrow shows the nodule deeply infiltrating the Douglas pouch and the anterior wall of the lower rectum. (*B*) T2W fat sat and (*C*) T1W fat sat sequences: it is possible to observe that the nodule (*arrow*) is completely hypointense in T1W scan.

190 had rectosigmoid endometriosis) showed that MR imaging has a sensibility of 85%, a specificity of 96%, a positive likelihood ratio (LR+) of 20.4, and a negative likelihood ratio (LR−) of 0.16 in diagnosing rectosigmoid endometriosis.[54] The major limitation of this metanalysis was that the prevalence of DE in the studies ranged from 6% to 76%, thus representing a significant heterogeneity. Another recent systematic

review and metanalysis on 8 studies (1132 patients) confirmed the diagnostic performance of MR imaging in diagnosing rectosigmoid endometriosis, reporting a sensitivity of 90%, a specificity of 96%, an LR+ of 17.26, and LR− of 0.15.[55]

3T MR imaging guarantees high spatial and contrast resolution. Its use has been studied in the diagnosis of DE.[56,57] In a prospective study,

46 women underwent a 3.0 T MR imaging examination with the following protocol: T2-weighted FrFSE HR sequences, T2-weighted FrFSE HR CUBE 3D sequences, T1-weighted FSE sequences, LAVA-flex sequences. The sensibility in diagnosing endometriosis was 96.97%, the specificity was 100.00%, the PPV was 100.00%, and the NPV was 92.86%.[56] A more recent retrospective study including 37 women investigated the diagnostic performance of 3.0 T MR imaging without intestinal hypotonization and rectal opacification in the diagnosis of DE. The authors reported a sensitivity of 94.4%, a specificity of 94.7%, PPV of 94.4%, and NPV of 95.0% for diagnosing rectosigmoid endometriosis.[57]

MR IMAGING ENEMA TECHNIQUE

DE can be difficult to distinguish from the surrounding structures because of its fibrous content. Given this background, rectosigmoid opacification with ultrasound gel can help to delineate the intestinal wall[47] and to identify intestinal endometriotic nodules (**Figs. 4–6**).[46,47] The retrograde distention is performed after the

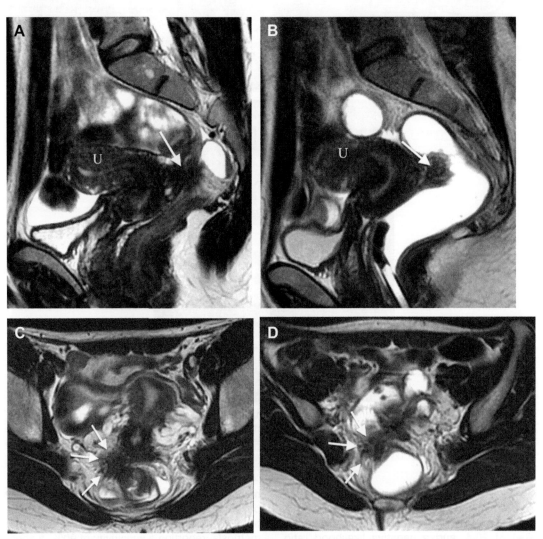

Fig. 4. (*A*) Fast relaxation FSE (FrFSE) T2W sequence without rectosigmoid enema: the nodule (*arrow*) is partially detectable and the rectal infiltration cannot be evaluated. (*B*) Sagittal FrFSE T2W sequence after distension: the endometriotic nodule is evident (*arrow*) and the infiltration of the anterior wall of the low rectum can be easily detected (U, uterus). (*C*) Axial FrFSE T2W sequences without distension rectal distension and (*D*) with rectal distension: the nodule is better detected after distension and it is surrounded by an intense desmoid reaction (*white arrows*).

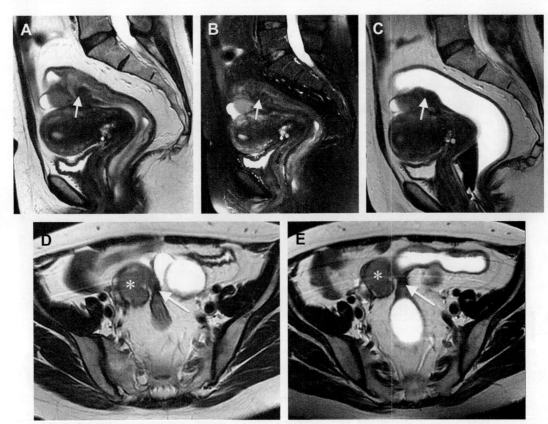

Fig. 5. A 29-year-old woman affected by dysmenorrhea and pelvic chronic pain. (*A, B*) FrFSE T2W and T2W fat sat sequences, sagittal plane. The intestinal nodule is not well detectable (*arrow*). (*C*) FrFSE T2W image with MR-enema: the fluid dilates the rectosigmoid lumen and the nodule becomes well detectable (*arrow*). (*D*) FSE T2W axial scan without distension: an endometrioma is present (*asterisk*) and the intestinal nodule is not detectable (*arrow*). (*E*) FSE T2W axial scan after rectal fluid distension: the endometrioma remains evident (*asterisk*), but now the intestinal endometriotic nodule is well visible (*arrow*).

patient lies on the MR imaging bed. It is usually performed on the lateral decubitus and then on the supine position. In claustrophobic patients, the prone decubitus may be used; it is also useful to reduce abdominal respiratory movements. The quantity of ultrasonographic gel used to distend the rectosigmoid varies in different studies: from 300–400 mL[38] to 150–200 mL.[47,58,59] A bowel preparation is usually performed before MR-e.[38,58] In fact, without cleansing the colon, rectosigmoid distention and opacification may be insufficient for diagnosing endometriotic nodules.[59] To decrease the peristalsis and improve the quality of the images, the patients are requested to fast for at least 4 hours before examination. Some radiologists use an antiperistalsis agent at the beginning of the examination,[47,59–61] whereas others do not use intestinal hypotonization because of the small quantity of intraluminal contrast medium.[38,58] Rectosigmoid opacification is obtained by some authors using ultrasonographic gel and by other authors using ultrasonographic gel diluted with saline solution (1:8).[38,62] The use of ultrasonographic gel allows to fill the rectosigmoid without causing over distention. In contrast, the identification of bowel wall retraction, a sign of the presence of rectosigmoid endometriosis, is facilitated by using it. Several authors do not routinely use paramagnetic contrast medium during MR-e in patients with suspicion of endometriosis.[47,59] Rectosigmoid endometriotic lesions are fibro-muscular structures located within the normal intestinal muscularis propria. Because of these histologic characteristics, after contrast medium injection, endometriotic nodules often have a very similar enhancement to the normal intestinal wall (**Figs. 7** and **8**).

The rectosigmoid lumen distended with ultrasound gel appears as low-intensity T1 and high intensity T2 sequences, with a well-defined

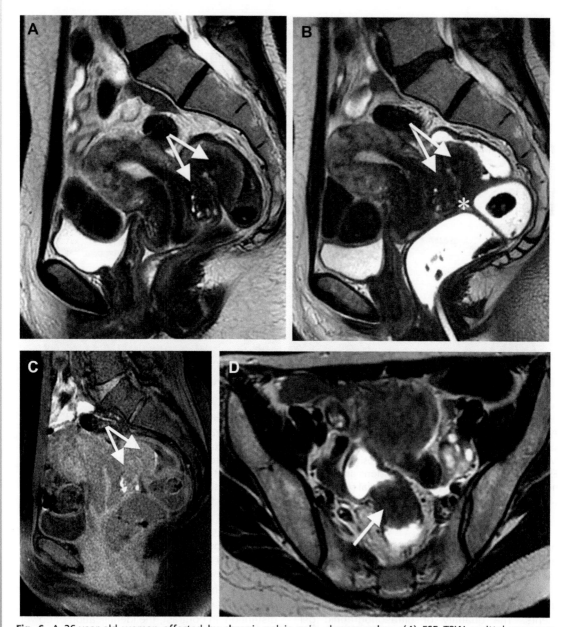

Fig. 6. A 26-year-old woman affected by chronic pelvic pain, dysmenorrhea. (*A*) FSE T2W sagittal sequence without rectal distension: The nodule (*arrows*) is poorly evident and the rectal wall is only partially evaluable. (*B*) FSE T2W sequence with rectum enema: the nodule is clearly evident (*arrows*), the Douglas pouch is obliterated (*asterisk*), and the muscularis propria of the anterior rectal wall is infiltrated. (*C*) FSE T1W sequence: the nodule (*arrow*) is usually hypointense because of its fibrous content. (*D*) Axial FSE T2W sequence: the endometriotic nodule is observed (*arrow*).

regular profile determined by the colonic wall (**Fig. 9**).[63] MR imaging does not allow to distinguish the different layers of the intestinal wall in the normal colon (serosa, muscularis propria, and mucosa).[47,59]

The occupation time of the scanner required to perform MR-e in patients with suspicion of DE ranges between 20[47] and 45 minutes.[38,62]

MR IMAGING ENEMA FINDINGS IN PATIENTS WITH RECTOSIGMOID ENDOMETRIOSIS

Few studies have described the use of MR-e in the diagnosis of rectosigmoid endometriosis. In a single-center prospective study, Chassang and colleagues[60] systematically opacified the rectum and the vagina with ultrasound gel to facilitate

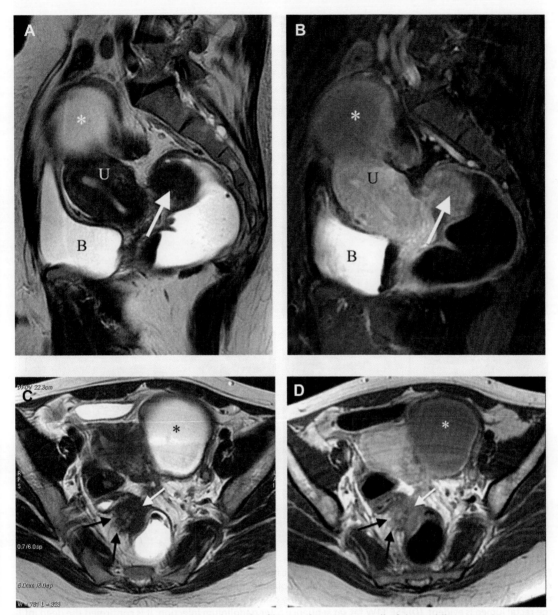

Fig. 7. (*A*) FrFSE T2W sequence: the nodule (*arrow*) infiltrates the anterior wall of the middle rectum (U, uterus; B, bladder). (*B*) FSE T1W fat sat sequence with injection of gadolinium: the contrast medium enhances the nodules, which is subperitoneal. (*C*) Axial FSE T2W and (*D*) FSE T1W sequences after gadolinium: the white arrows show the nodule that is causing a stenosis of the rectum. The rough margins of the nodule (*black arrows*) are determined by the desmoid reaction owing to endometriosis. In all images, an endometrioma (*asterisk*) is detectable.

the diagnosis of rectal and vaginal endometriotic nodules without using gadolinium-based contrast medium. The vagina was opacified with 60 mL of ultrasound gel and the rectum with 100 to 120 mL of gel. Images were obtained with a 1T MR imaging system using a phased array coil. Axial and sagittal T2-weighted images were performed both with and without vaginal and rectal opacification. Overall, 78 patients were included in the study; 31 had DE, of whom 24 were confirmed at laparoscopy; 17% had bowel endometriosis. Opacification significantly improved the sensitivity of MR imaging for the detection of DE (sensitivity: 63.1% without opacification and 81.7% with opacification). The specificity was excellent before (99.3%) and after opacification (100%). This study has some limitations: laparoscopy was not performed in all study patients, the

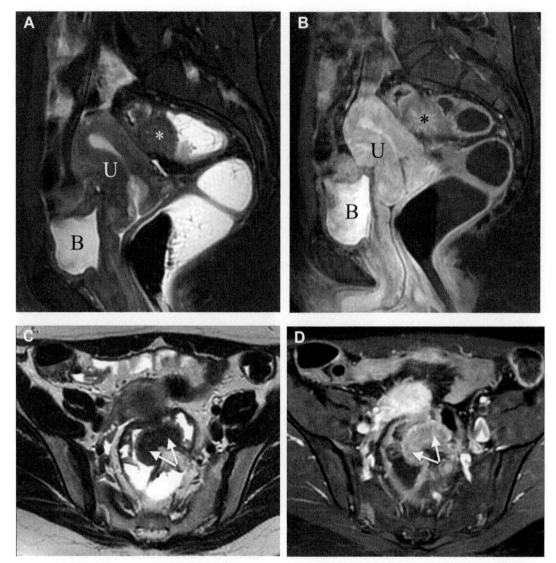

Fig. 8. (A) FrFSE T2W fat sat sequence: the endometriotic nodule deeply infiltrates the anterior wall of the higher rectum (*asterisk*). (B) FSE T1W fat sat sequence after gadolinium injection: the enhancement of the endometriotic nodule is shown. (C) Axial FSE T2W sequence: the nodule causes a distortion of the rectal wall and the stenosis of the rectal lumen is evident. (D) FSE T1W fat sat sequence after gadolinium injection: it is confirmed the deep infiltration of the rectal wall (U, uterus; B, bladder).

sample size was small, the prevalence of bowel endometriosis in the study population was low, and the authors used a 1.0 T magnet, which provides lower spatial resolution compared with the 1.5 T magnet, considered the standard magnetic field strength to be used in the diagnosis of endometriosis. A prospective study including 67 patients compared the performance of MR imaging realized without and with rectal and vaginal opacification for the diagnosis of vaginal and rectosigmoid endometriosis.[58] The opacification did not improve the performance of MR imaging in

diagnosing vaginal and rectosigmoid endometriosis. However, this finding was limited by the small number of patients with rectosigmoid endometriosis included in the study (23 out of 67).

Some studies compared MR-e with other imaging techniques used to diagnose endometriosis. A single-center prospective study compared the accuracy of MR-e and MDCT-e in diagnosing rectosigmoid endometriosis.[38] The study included 260 women, of whom 176 had surgical diagnosis of rectosigmoid endometriosis. There was no significant difference in the performance of the 2

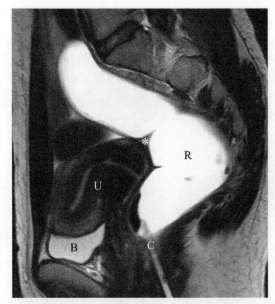

Fig. 9. Sagittal FSE T2W images: normal aspect of pelvic anatomy after rectosigmoid enema in a patient without endometriosis (B, bladder; U, uterus; asterisk, virtual Douglas pouch; R, dilated rectum; C, cannula for distension).

techniques in diagnosing rectosigmoid endometriosis (**Fig. 10**, **Table 1**). Both MDCT-e and MR-e underestimated the size of endometriotic nodules, and the underestimation was greater for nodules with largest diameter ≥30 mm. Moreover, MR-e was better tolerated by the patients compared with MDCT-e.

A single-center prospective study compared the performance of MR-e and TVS combined with water contrast in the rectum (named rectal water contrast TVS, RWC-TVS) in the diagnosis of rectosigmoid endometriosis.[62] The study included 286 patients, of whom 151 (52.8%) had rectosigmoid endometriosis at surgery. MR-e and RWC-TVS had similar performance in the diagnosis of rectosigmoid endometriosis (see **Table 1**). However, RWC-TVS performed better than MR-e in estimating the presence of the intestinal mucosa infiltration. MR-e and RWC-TVS underestimated the size of rectosigmoid endometriotic nodules compared with histology. Patients tolerated both radiologic techniques.

MR IMAGING: ENTEROGRAPHY AND COLONOGRAPHY

The main limitation of MR-e is that it allows to evaluate only the rectosigmoid colon. However, endometriosis may also affect other colonic tracts. This information is particularly important for patients

undergoing surgical treatment of bowel endometriosis because, if multicentric disease (multiple lesions affecting several bowel segments) is undiagnosed, the surgeon may not0 have the preoperative informed consent to treat all intestinal nodules. Therefore, the MR imaging evaluation of the whole colon has been proposed in the literature.

A prospective study including 33 patients showed that 3.0 T MR imaging and enterography can diagnose bowel endometriotic lesions located above the sigmoid.[64] The patients included in this study ingested a 5% mannitol solution (1000–1500 mL) 45 to 60 minutes before the examination. Intestinal hypotonization was performed. Small bowel and cecum distention were evaluated by performing balanced fast field-echo MR imaging sequences. Respiratory-triggered T2-weighted sequences and breath-hold 3D dual-echo Dixon sequences were performed before and after intravenous administration of contrast medium. Images of the upper and lower abdomen were acquired. 3.0 T MR imaging combined with enterography allowed to diagnose not only rectosigmoid endometriotic lesions but also nodules located on the ileum, ileocecal junction, cecum, appendix, and sigmoid colon. Two radiologists evaluated the MR imaging images. For the diagnosis of bowel nodules located above the rectosigmoid junction, MR imaging had an accuracy of 99.3% to 99.6%, a sensitivity of 92.3% to 96.2%, a specificity of 100%, a PPV of 100%, and an NPV of 99.3% to 99.6%.

Other studies investigated the role of contrast-enhanced MR-colonography (CE-MR-C) in the diagnosis of bowel endometriosis. This examination is performed after administering an antiperistaltic agent. A water enema of 1.5 to 2 L is administered using a 24 Foley rectal catheter. Intestinal distension is examined using a 2D thick slice (120 mm) RARE sequence (MR fluoroscopy). When complete colonic distension is achieved, contrast medium is administered intravenously. Two breath-hold sequences are launched with a delay of 60 seconds. The first group of sequences consists of axial, coronal, and sagittal THRIVE (T1W high resolution isotropic volume examination); the acquisition time is 19 seconds/sequence. The second group consists of axial, coronal and sagittal 2D balanced turbo-field echo; the acquisition time is 21 seconds/sequence. The diagnosis of bowel involvement is based on the presence of one or more of the following findings: nodule or plaque-like bowel wall thickening with hypointense signal on T2-weighted images and possible hyperintense foci on T1-weighted images with contrast enhancement after gadolinium injection;

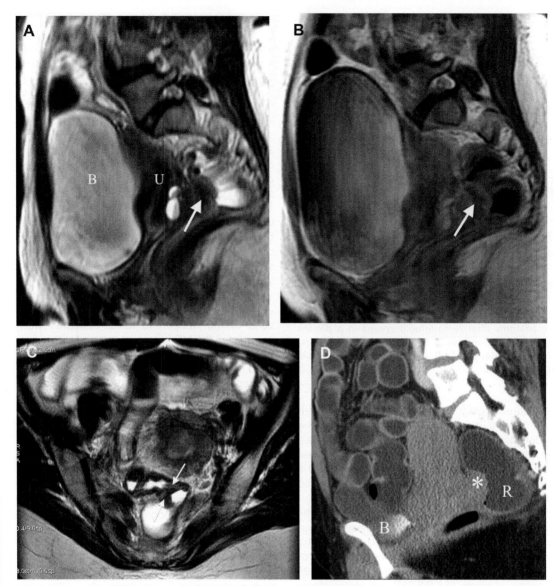

Fig. 10. MR-e and MDCT-enema examinations: a 23-year-old woman with deep dyspareunia and dysmenorrhea. (*A*) FSE T2W sequence: the arrow shows the rectal lesion (U, uterus; B, bladder). (*B*) FSE T1W sequence after gadolinium injection: poor enhancement of the endometriosis (*arrow*). (*C*) FrFSE T2W sequence: the lesion infiltrates the rectum (*arrow*). (*D*) MDCT-enema sagittal reconstruction (B, bladder; R, rectum). The asterisk shows the lesion infiltrating the anterior rectal wall.

loss of the fat tissue plane between the intestinal loop and the uterus or other adjacent organs; abnormal angulation of bowel loops. A prospective single-center study including 144 women with suspicion of endometriosis investigated the role of CE-MR-C for the diagnosis of intestinal endometriosis. The study protocol consisted of 2 phases. First, the patients underwent high-resolution MR imaging of the pelvis. Second, CE-MR-C of the entire colon was performed. Based on CE-MR-C images, sensitivity, specificity, PPV, NPV, and accuracy for diagnosis of colorectal endometriosis increased from 76%, 96%, 84%, 93%, and 91%, to 95%, 97%, 91%, 99%, and 97% for the most experienced radiologist (12 years' experience in genito-urinary imaging) and from 62%, 93%, 72%, 89%, and 85% to 86%, 94%, 82%, 96%, and 92% for the less experienced radiologist (2 years' experience). In particular, CE-MR-C was essential for diagnosing 2 cecal nodules.[65] A more recent study compared the diagnostic performance of TVS and

Table 1
Studies comparing the performance of MR-e and other imaging techniques in the diagnosis of rectosigmoid endometriosis

Authors	Imaging Technique	Accuracy (%)	Sensitivity (%)	Specificity (%)	PPV (%)	NPV (%)	LR+	LR−
Biscaldi et al,[38] 2014	MR-e	96.9	97.2	96.4	98.3	94.1	26.89	0.03
	MDCT-e	98.5	98.3	98.8	99.4	96.5	81.59	0.02
Leone Roberti Maggiore et al,[62] 2017	MR-e	96.5	95.4	97.8	98.0	95.0	42.91	0.05
	RWC-TVS	94.8	92.7	97.0	97.2	92.3	31.29	0.08

Abbreviations: LR+, positive likelihood ratio; LR−, negative likelihood ratio; NPV, negative predictive value; PPV, positive predictive value.

CE-MR-C in the diagnosis of DE.[66] The study included 90 patients of which 20 had bowel endometriosis. CE-MR-C allowed diagnosing of all cases of bowel endometriosis, including 1 case of ileal and 1 of cecal nodule that were not detected by TVS; overall, 100% correct diagnosis of bowel nodules, infiltration of the muscular layer and grade of stenosis were reported by the authors. The accuracy of TVS in diagnosing rectosigmoid nodules and in predicting the degree of infiltration was 91.1% and 88.9%, respectively. There was no significant difference between CE-MR-C and TVS in diagnosing rectosigmoid endometriosis and in predicting the degree of infiltration.

Compared with other imaging techniques used in the diagnosis of endometriosis, CE-MR-C has the advantage of visualizing the upper part of the colon and the small intestine. The main limitations of CE-MR-C are the need for bowel preparation and the length of the examination (about 30 minutes). Obviously, CE-MR-C requires the distention of the whole colon. A performing magnet (1.5 T or better 3 T) is mandatory to reduce the duration of the examination. Moreover, fast imaging is important because the colonic distention may be poorly tolerated by the patients.

SUMMARY

Noninvasive diagnosis of presence and characteristics of rectosigmoid endometriosis permits the best counseling of patients and thus ensures the best therapeutic planning. The main challenge in the diagnosis of rectosigmoid endometriosis is that these fibromuscular structures have a very close MR imaging signal to that of the surrounding healthy intestinal muscularis propria. As a consequence, rectal opacification with ultrasound gel after rectosigmoid cleansing helps to delineate the rectal wall and to identify endometriotic lesions. However, MR imaging cannot assess the depth of penetration of endometriosis in the intestinal wall. There is no evidence that the administration of paramagnetic contrast medium improves the diagnosis of rectosigmoid endometriosis. There is a need for multicentric studies with larger sample size to evaluate the reproducibility of MR-e in the diagnosis of rectosigmoid endometriosis for less experienced radiologists.

REFERENCES

1. Ferrero S, Arena E, Morando A, et al. Prevalence of newly diagnosed endometriosis in women attending the general practitioner. Int J Gynaecol Obstet 2010; 110(3):203–7.
2. Koninckx PR, Ussia A, Adamyan L, et al. Deep endometriosis: definition, diagnosis, and treatment. Fertil Steril 2012;98(3):564–71.
3. Remorgida V, Ferrero S, Fulcheri E, et al. Bowel endometriosis: presentation, diagnosis, and treatment. Obstet Gynecol Surv 2007;62(7):461–70.
4. Ferrero S, Camerini G, Ragni N, et al. Triptorelin improves intestinal symptoms among patients with colorectal endometriosis. Int J Gynaecol Obstet 2010;108(3):250–1.
5. Ferrero S, Camerini G, Venturini P, et al. Progression of bowel endometriosis during treatment with the oral contraceptive pill. Gynecol Surg 2011;8(3): 311–3.
6. Ferrero S, Camerini G, Ragni N, et al. Norethisterone acetate in the treatment of colorectal endometriosis: a pilot study. Hum Reprod 2010;25(1):94–100.
7. Ferrero S, Camerini G, Ragni N, et al. Letrozole and norethisterone acetate in colorectal endometriosis. Eur J Obstet Gynecol Reprod Biol 2010;150(2): 199–202.
8. Ferrero S, Barra F, Leone Roberti Maggiore U. Current and emerging therapeutics for the management of endometriosis. Drugs 2018;78(10):995–1012.
9. Ferrero S, Abbamonte LH, Remorgida V, et al. Irritable bowel syndrome and endometriosis. Eur J Gastroenterol Hepatol 2005;17(6):687.

10. Ferrero S, Camerini G, Ragni N, et al. Endometriosis and irritable bowel syndrome: co-morbidity or misdiagnosis? BJOG 2009;116(1):129 [author reply: 129–30].

11. Abrao MS, Goncalves MO, Dias JA Jr, et al. Comparison between clinical examination, transvaginal sonography and magnetic resonance imaging for the diagnosis of deep endometriosis. Hum Reprod 2007;22(12):3092–7.

12. Bazot M, Lafont C, Rouzier R, et al. Diagnostic accuracy of physical examination, transvaginal sonography, rectal endoscopic sonography, and magnetic resonance imaging to diagnose deep infiltrating endometriosis. Fertil Steril 2009;92(6):1825–33.

13. Barra F, Scala C, Biscaldi E, et al. Ureteral endometriosis: a systematic review of epidemiology, pathogenesis, diagnosis, treatment, risk of malignant transformation and fertility. Hum Reprod Update 2018;24(6):710–30.

14. Fedele L, Bianchi S, Portuese A, et al. Transrectal ultrasonography in the assessment of rectovaginal endometriosis. Obstet Gynecol 1998;91(3):444–8.

15. Alborzi S, Rasekhi A, Shomali Z, et al. Diagnostic accuracy of magnetic resonance imaging, transvaginal, and transrectal ultrasonography in deep infiltrating endometriosis. Medicine (Baltimore) 2018; 97(8):e9536.

16. Guerriero S, Condous G, Van den Bosch T, et al. Systematic approach to sonographic evaluation of the pelvis in women with suspected endometriosis, including terms, definitions and measurements: a consensus opinion from the International Deep Endometriosis Analysis (IDEA) group. Ultrasound Obstet Gynecol 2016;48(3):318–32.

17. Guerriero S, Ajossa S, Orozco R, et al. Accuracy of transvaginal ultrasound for diagnosis of deep endometriosis in the recto-sigmoid: systematic review and meta-analysis. Ultrasound Obstet Gynecol 2016;47(3):281–9.

18. Ferrero S, Scala C, Stabilini C, et al. Transvaginal ultrasonography with or without bowel preparation in the diagnosis of rectosigmoid endometriosis: prospective study. Ultrasound Obstet Gynecol 2019; 53(3):402–9.

19. Ferrero S, Leone Roberti Maggiore U, Barra F, et al. Modified ultrasonographic techniques. In: Guerriero S, Condous G, Alcazar JL, editors. How to perform ultrasonography in endometriosis. Springer; 2018. p. 133–45.

20. Dessole S, Farina M, Rubattu G, et al. Sonovaginography is a new technique for assessing rectovaginal endometriosis. Fertil Steril 2003;79(4):1023–7.

21. Valenzano Menada M, Remorgida V, Abbamonte LH, et al. Does transvaginal ultrasonography combined with water-contrast in the rectum aid in the diagnosis of rectovaginal endometriosis infiltrating the bowel? Hum Reprod 2008;23(5):1069–75.

22. Menada MV, Remorgida V, Abbamonte LH, et al. Transvaginal ultrasonography combined with water-contrast in the rectum in the diagnosis of rectovaginal endometriosis infiltrating the bowel. Fertil Steril 2008;89(3):699–700.

23. Reid S, Bignardi T, Lu C, et al. The use of intraoperative saline sonovaginography to define the rectovaginal septum in women with suspected rectovaginal endometriosis: a pilot study. Australas J Ultrasound Med 2011;14(3):4–9.

24. Reid S, Winder S, Condous G. Sonovaginography: redefining the concept of a "normal pelvis" on transvaginal ultrasound pre-laparoscopic intervention for suspected endometriosis. Australas J Ultrasound Med 2011;14(2):21–4.

25. Abrao MS, Neme RM, Averbach M, et al. Rectal endoscopic ultrasound with a radial probe in the assessment of rectovaginal endometriosis. J Am Assoc Gynecol Laparosc 2004;11(1):50–4.

26. Griffiths A, Koutsouridou R, Vaughan S, et al. Transrectal ultrasound and the diagnosis of rectovaginal endometriosis: a prospective observational study. Acta Obstet Gynecol Scand 2008;87(4): 445–8.

27. Delpy R, Barthet M, Gasmi M, et al. Value of endorectal ultrasonography for diagnosing rectovaginal septal endometriosis infiltrating the rectum. Endoscopy 2005;37(4):357–61.

28. Bahr A, de Parades V, Gadonneix P, et al. Endorectal ultrasonography in predicting rectal wall infiltration in patients with deep pelvic endometriosis: a modern tool for an ancient disease. Dis Colon Rectum 2006;49(6):869–75.

29. Bazot M, Bornier C, Dubernard G, et al. Accuracy of magnetic resonance imaging and rectal endoscopic sonography for the prediction of location of deep pelvic endometriosis. Hum Reprod 2007;22(5): 1457–63.

30. Kim A, Fernandez P, Martin B, et al. Magnetic resonance imaging compared with rectal endoscopic sonography for the prediction of infiltration depth in colorectal endometriosis. J Minim Invasive Gynecol 2017;24(7):1218–26.

31. Gordon RL, Evers K, Kressel HY, et al. Double-contrast enema in pelvic endometriosis. AJR Am J Roentgenol 1982;138(3):549–52.

32. Landi S, Barbieri F, Fiaccavento A, et al. Preoperative double-contrast barium enema in patients with suspected intestinal endometriosis. J Am Assoc Gynecol Laparosc 2004;11(2):223–8.

33. Faccioli N, Manfredi R, Mainardi P, et al. Barium enema evaluation of colonic involvement in endometriosis. AJR Am J Roentgenol 2008;190(4): 1050–4.

34. Savelli L, Manuzzi L, Coe M, et al. Comparison of transvaginal sonography and double-contrast barium enema for diagnosing deep infiltrating

endometriosis of the posterior compartment. Ultrasound Obstet Gynecol 2011;38(4):466–71.

35. Jiang J, Liu Y, Wang K, et al. Rectal water contrast transvaginal ultrasound versus double-contrast barium enema in the diagnosis of bowel endometriosis. BMJ Open 2017;7(9):e017216.

36. Biscaldi E, Ferrero S, Fulcheri E, et al. Multislice CT enteroclysis in the diagnosis of bowel endometriosis. Eur Radiol 2007;17(1):211–9.

37. Biscaldi E, Ferrero S, Remorgida V, et al. Bowel endometriosis: CT-enteroclysis. Abdom Imaging 2007;32(4):441–50.

38. Biscaldi E, Ferrero S, Leone Roberti Maggiore U, et al. Multidetector computerized tomography enema versus magnetic resonance enema in the diagnosis of rectosigmoid endometriosis. Eur J Radiol 2014;83(2):261–7.

39. Tzambouras N, Katsanos KH, Tsili A, et al. CT colonoscopy for obstructive sigmoid endometriosis: a new technique for an old problem. Eur J Intern Med 2002;13(4):274–5.

40. van der Wat J, Kaplan MD. Modified virtual colonoscopy: a noninvasive technique for the diagnosis of rectovaginal septum and deep infiltrating pelvic endometriosis. J Minim Invasive Gynecol 2007; 14(5):638–43.

41. Koutoukos I, Langebrekke A, Young V, et al. Imaging of endometriosis with computerized tomography colonography. Fertil Steril 2011;95(1): 259–60.

42. Jeong SY, Chung DJ, Myung Yeo D, et al. The usefulness of computed tomographic colonography for evaluation of deep infiltrating endometriosis: comparison with magnetic resonance imaging. J Comput Assist Tomogr 2013;37(5): 809–14.

43. van der Wat J, Kaplan MD, Roman H, et al. The use of modified virtual colonoscopy to structure a descriptive imaging classification with implied severity for rectogenital and disseminated endometriosis. J Minim Invasive Gynecol 2013;20(5): 543–6.

44. Mehedintu C, Brinduse LA, Bratila E, et al. Does computed tomography-based virtual colonoscopy improve the accuracy of preoperative assessment based on magnetic resonance imaging in women managed for colorectal endometriosis? J Minim Invasive Gynecol 2018;25(6):1009–17.

45. Ferrero S, Biscaldi E, Vellone VG, et al. Computed tomographic colonography vs rectal water- contrast transvaginal sonography in diagnosis of rectosigmoid endometriosis: a pilot study. Ultrasound Obstet Gynecol 2017;49(4):515–23.

46. Bazot M, Darai E, Hourani R, et al. Deep pelvic endometriosis: MR imaging for diagnosis and prediction of extension of disease. Radiology 2004; 232(2):379–89.

47. Loubeyre P, Petignat P, Jacob S, et al. Anatomic distribution of posterior deeply infiltrating endometriosis on MRI after vaginal and rectal gel opacification. AJR Am J Roentgenol 2009;192(6): 1625–31.

48. Qayyum A. Diffusion-weighted imaging in the abdomen and pelvis: concepts and applications. Radiographics 2009;29(6):1797–810.

49. Namimoto T, Awai K, Nakaura T, et al. Role of diffusion-weighted imaging in the diagnosis of gynecological diseases. Eur Radiol 2009;19(3): 745–60.

50. Moteki T, Ishizaka H. Diffusion-weighted EPI of cystic ovarian lesions: evaluation of cystic contents using apparent diffusion coefficients. J Magn Reson Imaging 2000;12(6):1014–9.

51. Ito TE, Abi Khalil ED, Taffel M, et al. Magnetic resonance imaging correlation to intraoperative findings of deeply infiltrative endometriosis. Fertil Steril 2017; 107(2):e11–2.

52. Guerriero S, Spiga S, Ajossa S, et al. Role of imaging in the management of endometriosis. Minerva Ginecol 2013;65(2):143–66.

53. Biscaldi E, Ferrero S, Remorgida V, et al. Rectosigmoid endometriosis with unusual presentation at magnetic resonance imaging. Fertil Steril 2009; 91(1):278–80.

54. Guerriero S, Saba L, Pascual MA, et al. Transvaginal ultrasound vs magnetic resonance imaging for diagnosing deep infiltrating endometriosis: systematic review and meta-analysis. Ultrasound Obstet Gynecol 2018;51(5):586–95.

55. Mourad J, Burke YZ. Needleless robotic-assisted abdominal cerclage in pregnant and nonpregnant patients. J Minim Invasive Gynecol 2016;23(3): 298–9.

56. Manganaro L, Fierro F, Tomei A, et al. Feasibility of 3.0T pelvic MR imaging in the evaluation of endometriosis. Eur J Radiol 2012;81(6):1381–7.

57. Yap SZL, Leathersich S, Lu J, et al. Pelvic MRI staging of endometriosis at 3T without patient preparation or anti-peristaltic: diagnostic performance outcomes. Eur J Radiol 2018;105:72–80.

58. Uyttenhove F, Langlois C, Collinet P, et al. Deep infiltrating endometriosis: should rectal and vaginal opacification be systematically used in MR imaging? Gynecol Obstet Fertil 2016;44(6):322–8.

59. Loubeyre P, Copercini M, Frossard JL, et al. Pictorial review: rectosigmoid endometriosis on MRI with gel opacification after rectosigmoid colon cleansing. Clin Imaging 2012;36(4):295–300.

60. Chassang M, Novellas S, Bloch-Marcotte C, et al. Utility of vaginal and rectal contrast medium in MRI for the detection of deep pelvic endometriosis. Eur Radiol 2010;20(4):1003–10.

61. Bazot M, Thomassin I, Hourani R, et al. Diagnostic accuracy of transvaginal sonography for deep

pelvic endometriosis. Ultrasound Obstet Gynecol 2004;24(2):180–5.

62. Leone Roberti Maggiore U, Biscaldi E, Vellone VG, et al. Magnetic resonance enema vs rectal water-contrast transvaginal sonography in diagnosis of rectosigmoid endometriosis. Ultrasound Obstet Gynecol 2017;49(4):524–32.

63. Coutinho A Jr, Bittencourt LK, Pires CE, et al. MR imaging in deep pelvic endometriosis: a pictorial essay. Radiographics 2011;31(2):549–67.

64. Rousset P, Peyron N, Charlot M, et al. Bowel endometriosis: preoperative diagnostic accuracy of 3.0-T MR enterography–initial results. Radiology 2014;273(1):117–24.

65. Scardapane A, Bettocchi S, Lorusso F, et al. Diagnosis of colorectal endometriosis: contribution of contrast enhanced MR-colonography. Eur Radiol 2011;21(7):1553–63.

66. Vimercati A, Achilarre MT, Scardapane A, et al. Accuracy of transvaginal sonography and contrast-enhanced magnetic resonance-colonography for the presurgical staging of deep infiltrating endometriosis. Ultrasound Obstet Gynecol 2012;40(5):592–603.

Rectal Cancer: Staging

Luís Curvo-Semedo, MD, PhD

KEYWORDS

- Rectal cancer • Magnetic resonance imaging • Staging • Structured report • Prognostic factors

KEY POINTS

- Primary staging by MR imaging is the cornerstone for decisions on the administration of neoadjuvant therapy and on the surgical procedure of choice in rectal cancer.
- Routine MR protocol should include high-resolution T2-weighted sequences in 3 planes and a diffusion-weighted sequence with high b-value.
- MR imaging assesses prognostic factors such as depth of tumor invasion into and beyond the rectal wall, the presence lymph node metastases, extramural venous invasion, involvement of the mesorectal fascia, and invasion of the peritoneum.

INTRODUCTION

The prognosis of rectal cancer is strongly related to several factors that include the depth of tumor invasion into and beyond the bowel wall,[1] the number of lymph nodes involved with tumor,[2] extramural venous invasion (EMVI),[3] involvement of the mesorectal fascia (MRF),[4] and the invasion of the peritoneum.[5] Accurate preoperative assessment of these prognostic factors is fundamental for selecting patients for neoadjuvant therapy and planning surgical approach to optimize complete excision.[6]

To improve patient selection for individually tailored therapies, accurate imaging techniques, able to differentiate early stage tumors from advanced tumors, are warranted. Several modalities have been used in the preoperative evaluation of rectal cancer, including endorectal ultrasound, computed tomography scans, and MR imaging.[7] However, a recent consensus paper stated that MR imaging should be the first-choice examination for primary staging of rectal cancer.[8] Because primary staging MR imaging needs to be as accurate as possible, the European Society of Gastrointestinal and Abdominal Radiology published a consensus paper on MR imaging for the clinical management of rectal cancer,[9] which was recently

updated,[10] with the aim of defining a state-of-the-art MR protocol for rectal cancer and how imaging findings should be interpreted and reported.

TECHNICAL NOTES AND PROTOCOL

MR imaging for staging rectal cancer should be performed with an external surface coil on a 1.5 T or 3.0 T MR imaging system. No consensus exists regarding the use of spasmolytics or endorectal filling for staging MR imaging examinations.[10] Spasmolytics can be beneficial for upper rectal tumors and when imaging is performed at 3.0 T, because in these cases bowel movement artifacts are most prevalent. Endorectal filling can reduce susceptibility artifacts related to luminal gas during diffusion-weighted imaging (DWI). However, its use cannot be recommended, because rectal wall distension may interfere with interpretation of the distance between the tumor and the MRF.[11] Another potential drawback of rectal filling is that the high T2 signal of the gel may originate shine-through effects on DWI. A potential alternative is the use of a microenema to reduce the amount of luminal gas.[12]

The protocol should include 2-dimensional high-resolution T2-weighted sequences in 3 planes. The axial and coronal images should be angulated

Disclosures: No disclosures to report.
University Clinic of Radiology, University of Coimbra, Clinical Academic Centre of Coimbra, Azinhaga de Santa Comba, 3000-548 Coimbra, Portugal
E-mail address: curvosemedo@gmail.com

Magn Reson Imaging Clin N Am 28 (2020) 105–115
https://doi.org/10.1016/j.mric.2019.09.003
1064-9689/20/© 2019 Elsevier Inc. All rights reserved.

(Fig. 1), respectively, perpendicular and parallel to the long axis of the lesion and the slice thickness should be 3 mm or greater. For low rectal cancers, images axial and coronal to the anal canal may be helpful in defining invasion of the sphincteric complex. A DWI sequence (including at least a high b-value of ≥800) should be also included even if there is no evident benefit for DWI at primary staging, but because DWI improves the response assessment after CRT.[9] Fat-suppressed, T1-weighted and dynamic contrast-enhanced sequences are not routinely recommended because they offer no additional benefits.[10]

Early cancers considered for local excision should be evaluated by (additional) endorectal ultrasound, given its superior diagnostic performance for differentiating T1 from T2 tumors.[13]

MESORECTAL FASCIA STATUS

Some authors suggest that CRM status, in combination with nodal status, yields a better prognostic model than the TNM system.[14] Recently, it was reported that the CRM status is superior to the TNM system for assessing the risk of local recurrence, disease-free survival and overall survival.[15]

Addressing accurately the relationship between the tumor and the MRF, which determines the status of the circumferential resection margin (CRM), because the MRF corresponds with the dissection plane in total mesorectal surgery, is probably the most important task that MR imaging has to fulfill (Fig. 2). Because sometimes staging (particularly T staging and specifically the differentiation between T2 and T3 tumors) will not noticeably change the overall preoperative or operative management of the patients, the clinically pertinent benefit of MR imaging is the assessment of the distance from the tumor to the MRF, which is strongly predictive of local recurrence.[16]

MR imaging provides an accurate information about CRM status. Beets-Tan and colleagues[17] reported that the prediction of MRF involvement was addressed with excellent interobserver agreement, allowing an MR imaging disease-free distance of 5 and 6 mm to correspond with a histopathologic disease-free margin of 1 and 2 mm, respectively. Another study confirmed a high accuracy (95%) for prediction of CRM status.[18] Brown and colleagues[19] showed a 92% agreement between MR images and histologic findings for prediction of the CRM.

A recent study showed that a margin of 1 mm or less measured by MR imaging correlated accurately with pathologic CRM involvement and poor outcome. The rate of pathologic CRM positivity was 53% in the group with a margin of 1 mm or less defined by MR imaging, and decreased to 7% to 8% when the tumor distance to the MRF was greater than 1 mm but no more than 5 mm. The 5-year local recurrence rate for patients with CRM-positive disease on MR imaging using a cut-off 1 mm or less was 20%, compared with 4% to 8% in those with larger margins.[20]

Recently, the European Society of Gastrointestinal and Abdominal Radiology consensus paper proposed that the MRF is involved if the distance between MRF and tumor is 1 mm or less, threatened if that distance is between 1 mm and 2 mm, and free if greater than 2 mm[10] (Fig. 3).

T STAGING

Preoperative T staging of rectal cancer by imaging is a complex task. Even if the present T-staging system is sometimes used for clinical decision making, it does not discriminate between tumors with a wide CRM and tumors with a threatened or involved CRM. Although many of these tumors are classified in the same stage (T3), they have a wholly different risk for local recurrence.

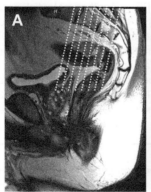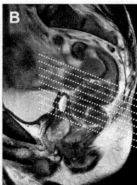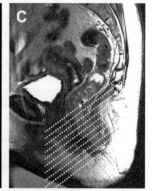

Fig. 1. Sagittal T2-weighted images showing the desired angulation of the axial images, perpendicular to the long axis of the neoplasm. (*A*) Upper third. (*B*) Middle third. (*C*) Lower third.

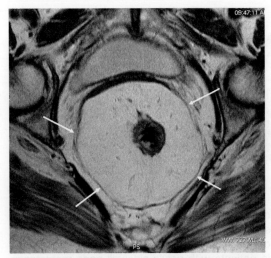

Fig. 2. Axial T2-weighted image depicting the MRF, appearing as a hypointense linear structure (*white arrows*) encircling the mesorectum.

The accuracy for T staging is not as high as desirable, varying between 65% and 86%[17,21–23] and was not as reproducible as expected, with considerable interobserver variability.[17] One exception to the above was shown by Brown and colleagues,[24] who reported 100% accuracy and complete agreement between 2 readers on the assessment of tumor stage.

Important MR imaging criteria relevant for T staging are summarized, according to Brown and colleagues,[19] as follows:

- Stage T1: low signal in the submucosa and replacement of the submucosal layer by abnormal signal not extending into the muscle coat
- Stage T2: intermediate signal within the muscularis propria
- Stage T3: broad-based bulge or nodular projection or intermediate signal projecting beyond outer muscle coat

- Stage T4: extension of abnormal signal into adjacent organ or through the peritoneal reflection

Therefore, the outer margin of the muscularis propria will remain intact with stage T2 tumors or less, whereas it will be disrupted in T3 disease (**Fig. 4**).

Nevertheless, most staging failures with MR imaging occur in the distinction between T2 stage and borderline T3 stage lesions,[17,24] with overstaging caused by desmoplastic reaction surrounding the lesions, because it is difficult to distinguish between spiculation in the perirectal fat caused by fibrosis alone (T2) and spiculation caused by fibrosis that contains tumor (T3).[17] Underestimation is less frequent and generally related to microscopic invasion of the mesorectal fat[25] (**Fig. 5**).

However, differentiating between minimal T3 infiltration and T2 lesions is probably of little consequence for patient management, because patients with minimal T3 infiltration into the mesorectal fat are also at low risk of surgical failure from CRM involvement.[26]

Conversely, the depth of tumor invasion is known to be an important prognostic factor, and the prognostic heterogeneity of T3 disease has been recognized previously.[26–28] In the Erlangen Registry of Colorectal Carcinomas, patients with cancer invading beyond the border of the muscularis propria by 5 mm or less had a significantly more favorable prognosis than those with invasion of more than 5 mm regarding local recurrence and cancer-related survival. Also, some pT3 patients had results like pT2 patients: for node-negative pT3 patients with invasion beyond the muscularis propria of 5 mm or less of and for node-negative pT2 patients, the local recurrence rates were 10% and 9%, with 5-year survival rates of 91% and 94%, respectively.[29]

Perhaps more important than defining the exact T3 substage based in the depth of invasion

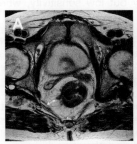
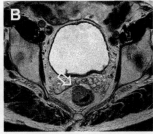
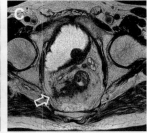

Fig. 3. Examples of the relation between the tumor and the MRF on axial T2-weighted images. (*A*) The margin is wide (*double arrow*) and the MRF is free (>2 mm). (*B*) The MRF is threatened because the margin is between 1 mm and 2 mm (*open arrow*). (*C*) The MRF is invaded because the tumor is contacting it (*open arrow*).

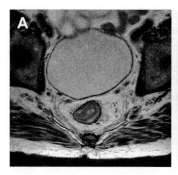
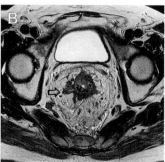

Fig. 4. Axial T2-weighted images of 2 patients. In (*A*) there is integrity of the hypointense muscular layer (T2 disease) whereas in (*B*) the tumor extends beyond muscularis propria into the mesorectal fat (maximal extension at 9 o'clock, *open arrow*), corresponding with T3 disease.

beyond the muscularis propria (T3a: <1 mm; T3b: 1–5 mm; T3c: 6–15 mm; T3d: >15 mm), is to differentiate tumors that, generally, could be approached primarily by surgery (T3a-b disease) from more advanced tumors (T3c-d disease) that should undergo preoperative (chemo)radiation therapy[30] (**Fig. 6**).

Stage T4 tumors are diagnosed by demonstrating infiltration into the peritoneal reflection (T4a) or adjacent organs (T4b) (**Fig. 7**).

N STAGING

Nodal disease is a powerful prognostic indicator. In the Dutch total mesorectal trial, patients with stage III (TxN1) disease had a 10-fold higher risk for local recurrence than did those with stage I (T1–2N0 stage) disease and a 3-fold higher risk than did those with stage II (T3N0 stage) disease.[31] Additionally, patients with stage N2 disease have a significantly higher risk of local recurrence compared with those with N0 or N1 disease.[32]

Rectal cancer most frequently spreads to the mesorectal lymph nodes, and, to a lesser degree, along the superior rectal artery.[33,34] Most mesorectal nodes are found at the level of the primary tumor.[35] The likelihood of nodal metastases increases with the T stage of the tumor, occurring in up to 50% of patients with stage T4 disease.[36]

Lateral pelvic sidewall nodal dissemination occurs in 10% to 25% of patients with rectal

cancer,[37] more often in low cancers.[38,39] Involved sidewall nodes increase the risk of systemic dissemination.[38] Predictably, the 5-year survival in patients with pelvic sidewall node metastases is low (25%–42%).[40] Because pelvic sidewall nodes are not routinely removed during total mesorectal surgery, extended lymphadenectomy may be needed.[41]

Only approximately 65% of mesorectal nodes found on histopathology can be identified on MR imaging.[42] Despite the identification of nodes as small as 2 to 3 mm, reliable detection of nodal metastases on MR imaging is currently not possible. The dilemma with enlarged nodes is to discriminate between reactive and metastatic nodes, and with small nodes micrometastases are easily missed.[43]

There has been limited success in the application of size criteria to characterize nodal disease, mainly because mesorectal nodes, whether benign or malignant, tend to be small. In a study of 424 surgical specimens containing 12,759 nodes, the mean nodal diameter was 3.34 mm and the mean diameter of metastasis was 3.84 mm.[33]

Moreover, there is no consensus on the size criterion for prediction of metastatic nodes. In previous studies, MR imaging size criteria were variable, ranging from any detectable node to nodes more than 1 cm. A higher cutoff value yields high specificity but low sensitivity, whereas the

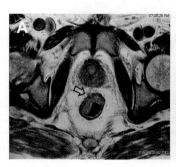
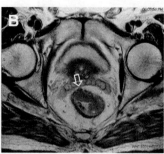

Fig. 5. Axial T2-weighted images of 2 patients with rectal cancers staged as (*A*) pT2 and (*B*) borderline pT3. A considerable similarity of the MR appearance of both tumors is noted, including a slight irregularity of the rectal wall owing to desmoplasia (*open arrow, A*) and minimal invasion beyond the muscularis propria (*open arrow, B*).

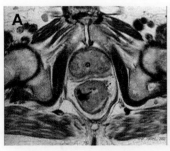
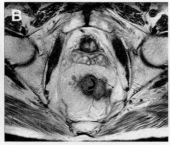

Fig. 6. Axial T2-weighted images of 2 patients with T3 disease. In (*A*), the depth of invasion beyond the muscularis propria is less than 5 mm (*double arrow*, 1 o'clock) indicating T3a-b disease, whereas in (*B*) the extramural disease is >5 mm (*double arrow*, 3–4 o'clock) representing T3c-d disease.

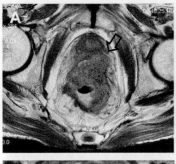
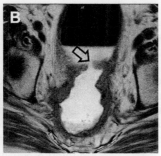
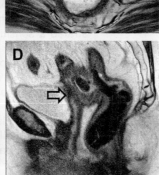

Fig. 7. T2-weighted images of patients with rectal cancers staged as T4b (*open arrows*). (*A*) Invasion of the prostate. (*B*) Invasion of the bladder with a rectovesical fistula. (*C*) Invasion of the sacrum. (*D*) Invasion of the vaginal dome.

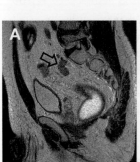
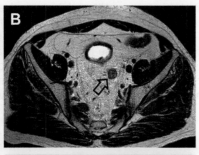
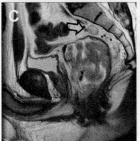
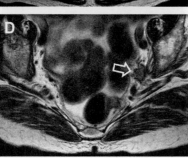

Fig. 8. T2-weighted images showing metastatic lymph nodes (*open arrows*). (*A*) A large node with irregular borders. (*B*) A large, round, heterogeneous node (*C*) A mucinous node with high signal. (*D*) A pelvic sidewall node with irregular margins and heterogeneous signal.

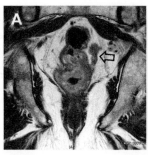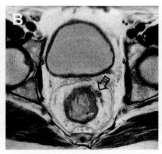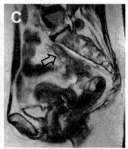

Fig. 9. (*A–C*) T2-weighted images of 3 patients with rectal cancer. There is tumoral signal intensity within the vascular structures, associated with irregular, nodular borders, and expansion of the vessel lumen (*open arrows*).

reverse is true if a smaller cutoff is used. The citations of long or short axis diameter were also unclear in most articles and the accuracy ranged widely (43%–85%).[21,23,44–53]

The borders and the signal characteristics of nodes on MR imaging seem more accurate than size in discriminating between benign and malignant nodes.[54,55] These are round-shaped, show irregular borders or display heterogeneous signal on T2-weighted images (**Fig. 8**).

Irregular nodal outline or signal heterogeneity, if present, resulted in a sensitivity of 85% and a specificity of 97% for detecting metastases in nodes 3 mm or greater.[54] However, in a study by Kim and colleagues,[55] spiculated and indistinct nodal borders on T2-weighted images were found to have 45% and 36% sensitivity, respectively, but 100% specificity.

The European Society of Gastrointestinal and Abdominal Radiology consensus paper proposed a combination of size and morphologic criteria to evaluate nodal disease, as follows: nodes with a short axis diameter 9 mm or greater are considered malignant; if nodal short axis diameter is 5 to 8 mm, the node should also have at least 2 morphologic criteria (round shape, irregular border, heterogeneous signal) to be malignant; for nodes less than 5 mm, all 3 morphologic criteria need to be present to consider the node involved; all mucinous nodes should be interpreted as malignant, irrespective of size. These criteria are applicable also to extramesorectal nodes.[10]

Owing to the lack of accuracy demonstrated by the conventional imaging methods, functional imaging has been explored for nodal characterization. MR imaging with ultrasmall superparamagnetic iron oxides showed promising results for nodal staging.[56,57] A Dutch study demonstrated a sensitivity of 93% and a specificity of 96%.[58] Another study could not replicate such high values, reporting a sensitivity of 65% and specificity of 93%, but these numbers are higher than for morphologic MR imaging criteria.[56]

Gadofosveset-enhanced MR imaging also improved the diagnostic performance compared with standard MR imaging, based on the different enhancement pattern between normal and metastatic nodes.[59,60] The negative predictive values of more than 95% on a per lesion and more than 85% on a per patient basis were equivalent to those of previous reports with ultrasmall superparamagnetic iron oxide.[59]

Although high b-value DWI is sensitive for localizing nodes, its role in their characterization is unproven, with necrotic neoplastic nodes yielding false-negative results and reactive hyperplastic nodes causing false-positive cases.[61] Moreover, nonmetastatic nodes are highly cellular and may cause restricted diffusivity.

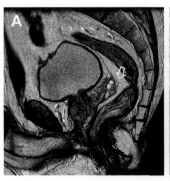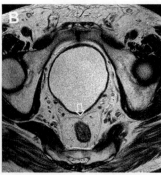

Fig. 10. T2-weighted images depicting the peritoneal reflection, connecting with the mid-rectum on the sagittal image (*open arrow on A*) and showing a "seagull" appearance on the axial plane (*open arrow on B*).

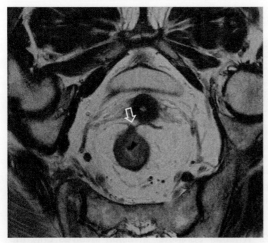

Fig. 11. Axial T2-weighted image of a patient with rectal cancer, displaying a nodular extension of intermediate signal (*open arrow*) through the fine hypointense peritoneal reflection above the level of its attachment to the anterior surface of the rectum.

EXTRAMURAL VENOUS INVASION

The presence of EMVI on MR imaging is associated with a 4-fold higher risk of distant metastasis (52% vs 12%), and a decrease in relapse-free survival at 3 years to only 35% versus 74% for patients without EMVI.[62]

By definition, EMVI is associated with tumors that are at least stage T3. MR imaging may display tumor invasion into the small noncharacterizable veins that radiate outward from the rectal wall, creating a nodular border. This can be differentiated from desmoplasia, which normally occurs as fine stranding. The presence of tumoral signal within a vascular structure is highly suggestive of EMVI: as a tumor invades along its lumen, the vessel expands; the tumor may grow through and beyond the vessel wall, disrupting it and producing an irregular or nodular border (**Fig. 9**). The sensitivity and specificity of MR imaging for detecting EMVI is around 62% and 88%, respectively.[63] Some patients with microscopic vascular invasion could not be resolved on MR imaging, whereas others with obvious EMVI on the preoperative images had false-negative histopathology owing to obliteration of normal venous architecture hampering the ability of the pathologist to recognize that a tumor deposit lies within a vessel.

PERITONEAL INVOLVEMENT

MR imaging can depict the location of the peritoneal reflection both on sagittal and axial images[64] (**Fig. 10**). The anterior peritoneal reflection separates the intraperitoneal and extraperitoneal portions of the mesorectal compartment; above the anterior peritoneal reflection, the mesorectal compartment is no longer enveloped by the MRF on its anterior aspect. Therefore, anterior MRF

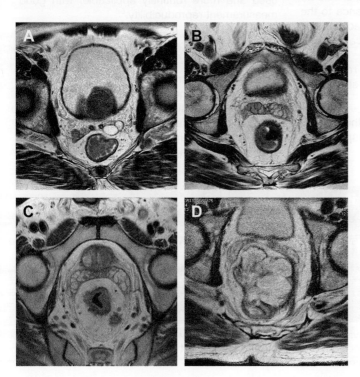

Fig. 12. T2-weighted images, showing tumors with different morphology. (*A*) A polypoid lesion. (*B*) A semiannular cancer. (*C*) An annular neoplasm (note, also a mesorectal tumor deposit at 4 o'clock). (*D*) A bulky tumor with high signal, corresponding with a mucinous cancer.

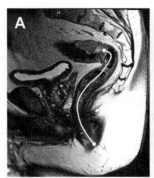
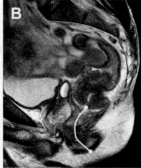
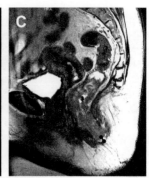

Fig. 13. Sagittal T2-weighted images displaying the measurement between the lower pole of the tumor and the anal verge. (*A*) Upper third. (*B*) Middle third. (*C*) Lower third.

involvement should only be reported below the level of the anterior peritoneal reflection.

The typical appearance of peritoneal involvement on MR imaging is shown in **Fig. 11**. The accuracy of MR imaging in correctly identifying peritoneal involvement is hampered by a failure to resolve microscopic infiltration of peritoneum.[65]

ADDITIONAL IMPORTANT INFORMATION

Additional information on rectal cancer MR imaging may be useful and should be included in the final report.[10]

Information about the morphology of the tumor, which includes its circumferential location within the rectal wall (eg, from X to X o'clock) should be reported (**Fig. 12**), as well as the distance to the anorectal junction or the anal verge, because this is fundamental to determine the surgical strategy (**Fig. 13**).

It is also essential to assess, for low rectal cancers, the degree of involvement of the sphincteric muscles (**Fig. 14**), by describing:

1. Whether the tumor invades only the internal sphincter or also involves the intersphincteric plane and external sphincter,

2. Whether sphincter invasion involves only the proximal one-third of the complex or extends into the middle and/or lower third, and

3. Whether the levator ani is involved.

Such information is pivotal when planning the surgical approach, particularly to determine if sphincter-saving resection is feasible without compromising local control. In such cases, an accurate anatomic description of the local extent is more informative than the T stage itself.[10]

Tumor size should be reported: even if tumor volume would probably be desirable, its determination is time consuming, and, from a practical standpoint, the tumor length is most commonly used and more routinely applicable, with good measurement reproducibility.[66]

STRUCTURED REPORTING

The implementation of structured report templates can improve the quality of MR imaging reporting for rectal cancer staging compared with free-text formats and leads to higher satisfaction levels from referring surgeons.[67] Therefore, their use should be encouraged.[10]

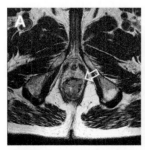
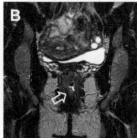
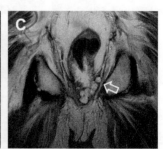

Fig. 14. T2-weighted images depicting invasion of the anal canal (*open arrows*). (*A*) Disruption of the internal sphincter with extension to the intersphincteric plane. (*B*) Invasion of the left internal and external sphincters. (*C*) Invasion of the left levator by a mucinous cancer.

SUMMARY

MR imaging has a pivotal role in the selection of patients with rectal cancer at different risk for local recurrence, because treatment is tailored according to the individual risk. As such, MR imaging is the preferred technique to stage this neoplasm. MR imaging assesses accurately the distance to the MRF, the degree of wall invasion, invasion of the surrounding organs and structures (including anal sphincter) and EMVI, therefore identifying ominous factors in patients who are at high risk for local recurrence. Nodal status assessment at present is still not very reliable.

REFERENCES

1. Harrison JC, Dean PJ, el-Zeky F, et al. From Dukes through Jass: pathological prognostic indicators in rectal cancer. Hum Pathol 1994;25:498–505.
2. Tang R, Wang JY, Chen JS, et al. Survival impact of lymph node metastasis in TNM stage III carcinoma of the colon and rectum. J Am Coll Surg 1995;180:705–12.
3. Talbot IC, Ritchie S, Leighton MH, et al. The clinical significance of invasion of veins by rectal cancer. Br J Surg 1980;67:439–42.
4. Adam IJ, Mohamdee MO, Martin IG, et al. Role of circumferential margin involvement in the local recurrence of rectal cancer. Lancet 1994;344:707–11.
5. Shepherd NA, Baxter KJ, Love SB. Influence of local peritoneal involvement on pelvic recurrence and prognosis in rectal cancer. J Clin Pathol 1995;48:849–55.
6. Barrett MW. Chemoradiation for rectal cancer: current methods. Semin Surg Oncol 1998;15:114–9.
7. Mathur P, Smith JJ, Ramsey C, et al. Comparison of CT and MRI in the pre-operative staging of rectal adenocarcinoma and prediction of circumferential margin involvement by MRI. Colorectal Dis 2003;5:396–401.
8. van de Velde CJ, Boelens PG, Borras JM, et al. EURECCA colorectal: multidisciplinary management: European consensus conference colon & rectum. Eur J Cancer 2014;50(1):1.e1–34.
9. Beets-Tan RGH, Lambregts DMJ, Maas M, et al. Magnetic resonance imaging for the clinical management of rectal cancer patients: recommendations from the 2012 European Society of Gastrointestinal and Abdominal Radiology (ESGAR) consensus meeting. Eur Radiol 2013;23(9):2522–31.
10. Beets-Tan RGH, Lambregts DMJ, Maas M, et al. Magnetic resonance imaging for clinical management of rectal cancer: updated recommendations from the 2016 European Society of Gastrointestinal and Abdominal Radiology (ESGAR) consensus meeting. Eur Radiol 2018;28(4):1465–75.
11. Slater A, Halligan S, Taylor SA, et al. Distance between the rectal wall and mesorectal fascia measured by MRI: effect of rectal distension and implications for preoperative prediction of a tumour-free circumferential resection margin. Clin Radiol 2006;61:65–70.
12. Van Griethuysen J, Bus E, Hauptmann M, et al. Air artefacts on diffusion-weighted MRI of the rectum: effect of applying a rectal micro-enema. Insights Imaging 2017;8(Suppl 1):S187.
13. Bipat S, Glas AS, Slors FJ, et al. Rectal cancer: local staging and assessment of lymph node involvement with endoluminal US, CT, and MRI—a meta-analysis. Radiology 2004;232:773–83.
14. Nagtegaal ID, Gosens MJ, Marijnen CA, et al. Combinations of tumor and treatment parameters are more discriminative for prognosis than the present TNM system in rectal cancer. J Clin Oncol 2007;25:1647–50.
15. Taylor FG, Quirke P, Heald RJ, et al. Preoperative magnetic resonance imaging assessment of circumferential resection margin predicts disease-free survival and local recurrence: 5-year follow-up results of the MERCURY study. J Clin Oncol 2014;32(1):34–43.
16. Nagtegaal ID, Quirke P. What is the role for the circumferential margin in the modern treatment of rectal cancer? J Clin Oncol 2008;26:303–12.
17. Beets-Tan RG, Beets GL, Vliegen RF, et al. Accuracy of magnetic resonance imaging in prediction of tumor-free resection margin in rectal cancer surgery. Lancet 2001;357:497–504.
18. Bissett IP, Fernando CC, Hough DM, et al. Identification of the fascia propria by magnetic resonance imaging and its relevance to preoperative assessment of rectal cancer. Dis Colon Rectum 2001;44:259–65.
19. Brown G, Radcliffe AG, Newcombe RG, et al. Preoperative assessment of prognostic factors in rectal cancer using high-resolution magnetic resonance imaging. Br J Surg 2003;90:355–64.
20. Taylor FGM, Quirke P, Heald RJ, et al. One millimetre is the safe cut-off for magnetic resonance imaging prediction of surgical margin status in rectal cancer. Br J Surg 2011;98:872–9.
21. Blomqvist L, Machado M, Rubio C, et al. Rectal tumor staging: MR imaging using pelvic phased-array and endorectal coils vs endoscopic ultrasonography. Eur Radiol 2000;10:653–60.
22. Blomqvist L, Holm T, Rubio C, et al. Rectal tumors: MR imaging with endorectal and/or phased-array coils, and histopathological staging on giant sections—a comparative study. Acta Radiol 1997;38:437–44.
23. Gagliardi G, Bayar S, Smith R, et al. Preoperative staging of rectal cancer using magnetic resonance imaging with external phase-arrayed coils. Arch Surg 2002;137:447–51.

24. Brown G, Richards CJ, Newcombe RG, et al. Rectal carcinoma: thin section MRI for staging in 28 patients. Radiology 1999;211:215–22.

25. Akasu T, Iinuma G, Fujita T, et al. Thin-section MRI with a phased-array coil for preoperative evaluation of pelvic anatomy and tumor extent in patients with rectal cancer. AJR Am J Roentgenol 2005;184:531–8.

26. Cawthorn SJ, Parums DV, Gibbs NM, et al. Extent of mesorectal spread and involvement of lateral resection margin as prognostic factors after surgery for rectal cancer. Lancet 1990;335:1055–9.

27. Park YJ, Youk EG, Choi HS, et al. Experience of 1446 rectal cancer patients in Korea and analysis of prognostic factors. Int J Colorectal Dis 1999;14:101–6.

28. Willett CG, Badizadegan K, Ancukiewicz M, et al. Prognostic factors in stage T3N0 rectal cancer: do all patients require postoperative pelvic irradiation and chemotherapy? Dis Colon Rectum 1999;42:167–73.

29. Merkel S, Mansmann U, Siassi M, et al. The prognostic inhomogeneity in pT3 rectal carcinomas. Int J Colorectal Dis 2001;16:298–304.

30. Glynne-Jones R, Wyrwicz L, Tiret E, et al. Rectal cancer: ESMO Clinical Practice Guidelines for diagnosis, treatment and follow-up. Ann Oncol 2017;28(Supplement 4):iv22–40.

31. Kapiteijn E, Marijnen CA, Nagtegaal ID, et al. Preoperative radiotherapy combined with total mesorectal excision for resectable rectal cancer. N Engl J Med 2001;345:638–46.

32. Moran MR, James EC, Rothenberger DA, et al. Prognostic value of positive lymph nodes in rectal cancer. Dis Colon Rectum 1992;35:579–81.

33. Dworak O. Morphology of lymph nodes in the resected rectum of patients with rectal carcinoma. Pathol Res Pract 1991;187:1020–4.

34. Steup WH, Moriya Y, van de Velde CJ. Patterns of lymphatic spread in rectal cancer. A topographical analysis on lymph node metastases. Eur J Cancer 2002;38:911–8.

35. Koh DM, Brown G, Temple L, et al. Distribution of mesorectal lymph nodes in rectal cancer: in vivo MR imaging compared with histopathological examination. Initial observations. Eur Radiol 2005;15:1650–7.

36. Hida J, Yasutomi M, Maruyama T, et al. Lymph node metastases detected in the mesorectum distal to carcinoma of the rectum by the clearing method: justification of total mesorectal excision. J Am Coll Surg 1997;184:584–8.

37. Hojo K, Koyama Y, Moriya A, et al. Lymphatic spread and its prognostic value in patients with rectal cancer. Am J Surg 1982;144:350–4.

38. Hocht S, Mann B, Germer CT, et al. Pelvic sidewall involvement in recurrent rectal cancer. Int J Colorectal Dis 2004;19:108–13.

39. Ueno H, Mochizuki H, Hashiguchi Y, et al. Prognostic determinants of patients with lateral nodal involvement by rectal cancer. Ann Surg 2001;234:190–7.

40. Hida J, Yasutomi M, Fujimoto K, et al. Does lateral lymph node dissection improve survival in rectal cancer? Examination of node metastases by the clearing method. J Am Coll Surg 1997;184:475–80.

41. Suzuki K, Muoto T, Sawada T. Prevention of local recurrence by extended lymphadenectomy for rectal cancer. Surg Today 1995;25:795–801.

42. Koh DM, Brown G, Husband JE. Nodal staging in rectal cancer. Abdom Imaging 2006;31:652–9.

43. Dworak O. Number and size of lymph nodes and node metastases in rectal carcinomas. Surg Endosc 1989;3:96–9.

44. Vogl TJ, Pegios W, Mack MG, et al. Accuracy of staging rectal tumors with contrast-enhanced transrectal MR imaging. AJR Am J Roentgenol 1997;168:1427–34.

45. Maier AG, Kersting-Sommerhoff B, Reeders JW, et al. Staging of rectal cancer by double-contrast MR imaging using the rectally administered superparamagnetic iron oxide contrast agent ferristene and IV gadodiamide injection: results of a multicenter phase II trial. J Magn Reson Imaging 2000;12(5):651–60.

46. Okizuka H, Sugimura K, Yoshizako T, et al. Rectal carcinoma: prospective comparison of conventional and gadopentetate dimeglumine enhanced fat-suppressed MR imaging. J Magn Reson Imaging 1996;6(3):465–71.

47. de Lange EE, Fechner RE, Edge SB, et al. Preoperative staging of rectal carcinoma with MR imaging: surgical and histopathologic correlation. Radiology 1990;176(3):623–8.

48. Blomqvist L, Rubio C, Holm T, et al. Rectal adenocarcinoma: assessment of tumour involvement of the lateral resection margin by MRI of resected specimen. Br J Radiol 1999;72(853):18–23.

49. Thaler W, Watzka S, Martin F, et al. Preoperative staging of rectal cancer by endoluminal ultrasound vs. magnetic resonance imaging. Preliminary results of a prospective, comparative study. Dis Colon Rectum 1994;37(12):1189–93.

50. Kusunoki M, Yanagi H, Kamikonya N, et al. Preoperative detection of local extension of carcinoma of the rectum using magnetic resonance imaging. J Am Coll Surg 1994;179(6):653–6.

51. Kim NK, Kim MJ, Park JK, et al. Preoperative staging of rectal cancer with MRI: accuracy and clinical usefulness. Ann Surg Oncol 2000;7(10):732–7.

52. Urban M, Rosen HR, Holbling N, et al. MR imaging for the preoperative planning of sphincter-saving surgery for tumors of the lower third of the rectum: use of intravenous and endorectal contrast materials. Radiology 2000;214(2):503–8.

53. Zerhouni EA, Rutter C, Hamilton SR, et al. CT and MR imaging in the staging of colorectal carcinoma: report of the Radiology Diagnostic Oncology Group II. Radiology 1996;200:443–51.

54. Brown G, Richards CJ, Bourne MW, et al. Morphologic predictors of lymph node status in rectal cancer with use of high spatial resolution MRI with histopathologic comparison. Radiology 2003;227: 371–7.

55. Kim JH, Beets GL, Kim MJ, et al. High-resolution MRI for nodal staging in rectal cancer: are there any criteria in addition to the size? Eur J Radiol 2004;52:78–83.

56. Koh DM, George C, Temple L, et al. Diagnostic accuracy of nodal enhancement pattern of rectal cancer at MRI enhanced with ultrasmall superparamagnetic iron oxide: findings in pathologically matched mesorectal lymph nodes. AJR Am J Roentgenol 2010;194:W505–13.

57. Koh DM, Brown G, Temple L, et al. Rectal cancer: mesorectal lymph nodes at MR imaging with USPIO versus histopathologic findings—initial observations. Radiology 2004;231:91–9.

58. Lahaye MJ, Engelen SM, Kessels AG, et al. USPIO-enhanced MR imaging for nodal staging in patients with primary rectal cancer: predictive criteria. Radiology 2008;246:804–11.

59. Lambregts DM, Beets GL, Maas M, et al. Accuracy of Gadofosveset-enhanced MRI for Nodal Staging and Restaging in Rectal Cancer. Ann Surg 2011; 253:539–45.

60. Lahaye MJ, Beets GL, Engelen SME, et al. Gadovosfeset trisodium (Vasovist ®) enhanced MR lymph node detection: initial observations. Open Magn Reson J 2009;2:1–5.

61. Figueiras RG, Goh V, Padhani AR, et al. The role of functional imaging in colorectal cancer. AJR Am J Roentgenol 2010;195(1):54–66.

62. Newland R, Dent O, Lyttle M, et al. Pathological determinants of survival associated with colorectal cancer with lymph node metastases. Cancer 1994; 73:2076–82.

63. Smith NJ, Shihab O, Arnaout A, et al. MRI for detection of extramural vascular invasion in rectal cancer. AJR Am J Roentgenol 2008;191:1517–22.

64. Gollub MJ, Maas M, Weiser M, et al. Recognition of the anterior peritoneal reflection at rectal MRI. AJR Am J Roentgenol 2013;200:97–101.

65. Brown G, Daniels IR. Preoperative staging of rectal cancer: the MERCURY research project. Recent Results Cancer Res 2005;165:58–74.

66. Hotker AM, Tarlinton L, Mazaheri Y, et al. Multiparametric MRI in the assessment of response of rectal cancer to neoadjuvant chemoradiotherapy: a comparison of morphological, volumetric and functional MRI parameters. Eur Radiol 2016;26:4303–12.

67. Norenberg D, Sommer WH, Thasler W, et al. Structured reporting of rectal Magnetic Resonance Imaging in suspected primary rectal cancer: potential benefits for surgical planning and interdisciplinary communication. Invest Radiol 2016;52:232–9.

Rectal Cancer
Assessing Response to Neoadjuvant Therapy

Monique Maas, MD, PhD[a],*, Rebecca A.P. Dijkhoff, MD[b],
Regina Beets-Tan, MD, PhD[a]

KEYWORDS

• Rectal cancer • MR imaging • Staging • Post-CRT evaluation

KEY POINTS

- Restaging after chemoradiation in rectal cancer is crucial for treatment planning.
- Main challenges are identification of a complete response, extent of residual tumor and nodal stage after CRT.
- Complete response detection is best performed by combining T2-weighted MR imaging, diffusion-weighted imaging, and endoscopy.
- Use of a structured report or checklist is recommended.

INTRODUCTION

Many patients with rectal cancer are treated with neoadjuvant chemoradiation. Generally, in the United States, patients who have cT3 to 4N0 or any TN+ disease are candidates for neoadjuvant chemoradiation. Proximal T3N0 tumors sometimes may proceed to immediate resection; however, nodal metastasis is present in up to 22% of these patients, possibly leading to undertreatment if chemoradiation is omitted.[1,2] The purpose of this neoadjuvant treatment is[1] to reduce tumor volume and stage to facilitate resection and[2] to decrease local recurrence rates. Chemoradiation usually consists of a 5-FU-based agent (eg, capecitabine) and is combined with 45.0 to 50.4 Gy of radiation in daily fractions on weekdays. Restaging of the tumor after chemoradiation is performed around 8 to 10 weeks after the last radiation dose. Downsizing occurs in the majority of patients and even complete disappearance of the tumor and involved nodes occurs in approximately 16% of

the patients (ypT0N0, complete response).[3] The purpose of restaging is to reassess resectability of the tumor and to determine whether surgical treatment can be potentially avoided in patients with a complete response. In this article, the restaging of rectal cancer after chemoradiation is discussed, in particular the role of MR imaging.

NORMAL ANATOMY AND IMAGING TECHNIQUES

After chemoradiation, the main anatomy of the rectum and mesorectum remains the same; however, changes in the rectal wall, mesorectum, and surrounding structures can be seen. Owing to the irradiation submucosal edema occurs, which makes the rectal wall layer appear thickened and 3-layered on MR imaging (contrasting to a 2-layered wall in the normal untreated rectum; **Fig. 1**). This is usually most prominently visible in the distal rectum. Within the mesorectum, fluid and edema can be seen as well and fluid in the

Disclosure Statement: The authors have nothing to disclose.
[a] Department of Radiology, The Netherlands Cancer Institute, PO Box 90203, Amsterdam 1006BE, the Netherlands; [b] Department of Internal Medicine, Zuyderland Medical Centre, PO Box 5500, 6130MB Sittard/Heerlen, the Netherlands
* Corresponding author.
E-mail address: m.maas@nki.nl

Magn Reson Imaging Clin N Am 28 (2020) 117–126
https://doi.org/10.1016/j.mric.2019.09.004

mri.theclinics.com

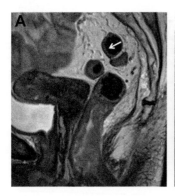 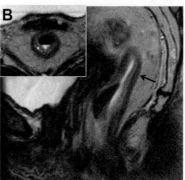

Fig. 1. (*A*) Before CRT, only 2 layers are visible in the wall. The slightly hyperintense mucosa (inner/luminal layer) and the outer muscular layer, which is hypointense. (*B*) After CRT, 3 layers are visible: the inner mucosal layer and muscular layer on the outside, but now a hyperintense layer is visible in between, which is the submucosa with edema. The inset in the upper left corner of B shows the axial view with an asterisk indicating the submucosal edema.

peritoneal reflection or along the mesorectal fascia is not an uncommon finding. Lymph nodes decrease in size (regardless of their metastatic status) and some disappear.[4]

Restaging of rectal cancer after chemoradiation is mostly performed with MR imaging, but endoscopic ultrasound imaging can be used as an adjunct, to assess whether there is still a yT1 or yT2 tumor, if local excision is considered. MR imaging has the advantage of depicting the whole rectum and mesorectum, including surrounding organs and nodes, whereas with endoscopic ultrasound imaging these structures can only partially be evaluated by the limited field of view (just as in primary staging of rectal cancer). Endoscopy is an important additional tool to assess response and specifically when an organ preserving strategy is considered, endoscopy is crucial to perform next to MR imaging.[5]

IMAGING PROTOCOL

For restaging after CRT, the same protocol can be used as for primary staging, consisting of T2-weighted sequences in 3 orthogonal directions (sagittal, coronal, and axial), where the axial plane is perpendicular to the (former) tumor axis and the coronal plane is parallel. An axial DWI (exact same angle as the axial T2-weighted sequence) is important in restaging after CRT (including a high b-value of 800–1000). The apparent diffusion coefficient (ADC) map must be constructed and send to the PACS. An unenhanced T1-weighted large field of view sequence can be considered to depict the whole regional lymph drainage route and it can be helpful to assess bony changes in some cases. If a large field of view T1 sequence is not used, the T2 sequence should be scanned with a large field of view. It is important to compare the post-CRT images with the pre-CRT MR imaging during MR imaging acquisition to identify the (former) tumor location, because, owing to tumor response, this can be challenging sometimes. For restaging

purposes use of an enema before the MR imaging has been shown to significantly decrease artifacts, which make the evaluation of DWI easier; therefore, the use of an enema is recommended. Ultrasound gel shows T2 shine through and is not recommended, because it obscures any residual high signal of tumor in the rectal wall.

Table 1 shows an example of an MR imaging protocol, as used in the authors' institution.

IMAGING FINDINGS AND DIAGNOSTIC CRITERIA

Most of the tumors will respond to chemoradiation and show a degree of response. For treatment purposes it is important to answer the following questions:

- Is there residual luminal tumor?
- If these is residual tumor, what is the ycT stage?
- Are there any findings that indicate a risk for incomplete resection?
- Is there (residual) nodal involvement?

Is There Residual Luminal Tumor?

As mentioned, many tumors show response. When a tumor responds to chemoradiation, tumor tissue is replaced by fibrosis. Fibrosis has a hypointense signal. The distribution of the fibrosis tends to follow the distribution of the tumor: that is, if the tumor was circular, the fibrosis will also be circular. Also, the shape will generally not change, for example, an irregular spiculated tumor will show irregular fibrosis as well. A complete response (ypT0) will show either a normalized rectal wall (rare, approximately 5% of cases with ypT0) or homogeneous fibrosis without diffusion restriction.[6] However, irregular more heterogeneous fibrosis or fibrosis with focal diffusion restriction sometimes do correspond with a complete response after surgery. The

Table 1
An example of an MR imaging protocol

	Sagittal T2 SE	Axial T2 SE	Coronal T2 SE	T1W	DWI
TR	3357	11,838	8456	9.8	2829
TE	150	130	130	4.6	95
NSA	3	2	2	1	8
Acquired in plane resolution (mm)	0.78 × 1.12	0.78 × 1.15	0.78 × 1.15	1.14 × 1.15	2.25 × 2.32
Matrix	256 × 178	256 × 174	256 × 174	264 × 261	80 × 65
Slice thickness (mm)	4	3	3	1	5
Slices	22	42	30	200	20
Time (min)	4:43	5:43	4:05	6:11	1:33
EPI factor					65
b-values					0, 1000
Fat suppression					SPIR

sensitivity of T2-weighted imaging for the prediction of a complete response is low (19%).[7] Patel and colleagues[8] recommended to use the mr tumour regression grade (mrTRG) system, which is a radiologic counterpart for the TRG system that is used in histopathology to grade response.[9] Essentially, the mrTRG is a method to assess the amount of fibrosis and residual tumor, which is very similar to but more standardized than standard evaluation of the response to CRT. Unfortunately, the sensitivity to detect a complete response is still only 74% when using mrTRG.[10] The addition of a DWI sequence increases overall diagnostic performance to 80%, when using the presence of absence of diffusion restriction as a diagnostic criterion. In these cases, sensitivity was reported to be rather disappointing (52%–64%), meaning that many complete responses are missed.[11] A more pattern-based approach has been proposed to improve diagnostic performance. Similar to the morphologic response at T2-weighted (TW2) MR imaging, response on diffusion tends to follow the shape of the tumor as well. Polypoid or semicircular tumors usually show focal diffusion restriction, whereas circular tumors have scattered areas of diffusion restriction or circular more massive diffusion restriction. By use of such a pattern-based approach, a sensitivity of 94% and specificity of 77% could be reached to predict complete response in experienced hands.[6] The results of this study are promising and can hopefully be reproduced in a prospective setting. **Fig. 2** shows an example of a complete response on T2W MR imaging and DWI.

During the last years a paradigm shift has occurred, where organ preservation is becoming increasingly considered in complete responders.[12–14] One of the main treatment determinants in organ preservation is endoscopy. Nowadays, endoscopy is an invaluable part of response assessment and follow-up. Maas and colleagues[5] have shown that to assess luminal response, endoscopy yields the highest diagnostic performance compared with T2-MR imaging and DWI. They also showed that when endoscopy, T2-MR imaging, and DWI all indicate that a tumor has responded completely the chance for a true complete response was 98%. So, when considering a wait-and-see policy, the combination of endoscopy and MR imaging is crucial.

Mucinous tumors and mucinous degeneration
Mucinous tumors show a much poorer response to chemoradiation than solid adenocarcinomas (**Fig. 3**). Usually, the solid part does show response to chemoradiation, whereas the mucinous part does not regress or will even progress.[15] Another entity is mucinous degeneration of a tumor, which is only present in a small subset of tumors. This mucinous degeneration can lead to small areas of high signal in the former tumor bed. When assessed by histology, such mucin lakes are usually acellular and might be a sign of a good response. However, another hypothesis is that small mucinous areas in the primary tumor have not responded to CRT and grew despite the CRT, which would correspond with partial response combined with progression or even

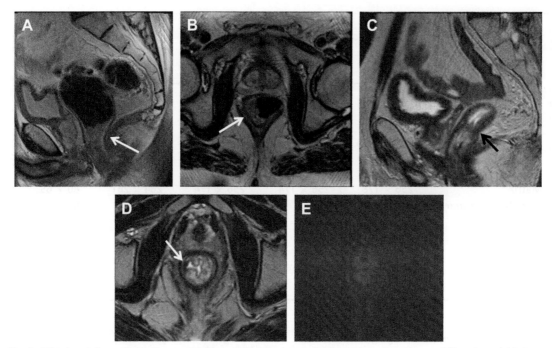

Fig. 2. Distal rectal cancer (*A, B, arrow*) before CRT that showed only a minor focal area of fibrosis and (*C, D, arrow*) after CRT, (*E*) without diffusion restriction, indicative of a complete response.

dedifferentiation of the tumor. The latter group, however, would probably have cellular mucin rather than acellular mucin at pathology.

What Is the ycT-Stage and Are There Risks for Incomplete Resection?

Depending on the residual ycT-stage treatment is determined. A small T1 tumor can possibly be treated with local excision, whereas higher T stages require a total mesorectal excision. In case of residual mesorectal fascia involvement or a T4b tumors, a more extensive resection is necessary. In distal tumors, the surgeon needs to decide on a very low anterior resection or abdominoperineal resection. MR imaging can be of help,

but this last decision is generally based on digital rectal examination.

Primarily, MR imaging will be performed after chemoradiation to assess tumor response. Just as in primary staging, MR imaging cannot distinguish a ycT1 tumor from a ycT2 tumor, so endoscopic ultrasound imaging is necessary to further evaluate this. MR imaging is accurate in predicting confinement of a tumor to the rectal wall (maximally ycT2) after CRT, with an area under the curve of 0.86.[16] The main issue is overstaging of residual tumor; that is, ycT2 tumors are mistaken as ycT3 tumors. This can be explained by the fact that mesorectal stranding in pretreatment cT3 tumors usually remain visible as thin fibrotic strands and to err on the safe side a

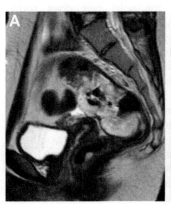
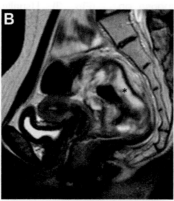

Fig. 3. (*A*) A mucinous tumor (*asterisk*) is visible before CRT. (*B*) After CRT, there is hardly any response.

radiologist tend to overestimate the amount of tumor in these strands. **Fig. 4** shows a tumor that has responded, but still had after ycT3ab tumor CRT. There is very limited evidence on the value of MR imaging to predict regression of cT4 tumors. The tumor invasion into other organs usually also shows a fibrotic transformation. If there is no diffusion restriction, the tumor has likely become less than ycT4, but during surgery the organ usually has to be resected anyway, because the fibrosis makes it impossible for surgeons to decide where to safely cut without causing an incomplete resection. In **Fig. 5**, a cT4 tumor is shown before and after CRT.

Regression of mesorectal fascia invasion can be challenging after CRT. At pretreatment staging, MR imaging is very accurate in determining MRF invasion, but owing to the appearance of fibrotic strands at former tumor invasion (similar to regression in cT3 tumors, as described elsewhere in this article) radiologists tend to overstage. Only when an intact fat plane becomes visible between tumor and MRF can one be certain that the MRF is no longer involved.

In distal tumors, regression from the anorectal junction is important to determine the feasibility of sphincter preservation. Surgeons generally evaluate this based on digital rectal examination, but MR imaging can be helpful. A study by Krdzalic and colleagues[17] showed that CRT causes an increase in the distance between lower tumor border and anorectal junction and that the measurement of this distance on MR imaging is associated with the ability to predict sphincter preservation.

Nodal Response

Nodal staging in rectal cancer is challenging and can be even more challenging after CRT. Size criteria are the basis for nodal staging, but these are unreliable because large nodes can be reactive and small nodes harbor metastases in up to 20% (nodes between 2 and 5 mm).[18] Addition of morphologic criteria (round shape, border irregularity, and heterogeneity in signal intensity) can improve accuracy, but still accuracies remain rather low. After CRT all nodes (both benign and malignant) decrease in size and approximately 44% will disappear.[4] Given the small size of nodes after CRT, morphology can be difficult to evaluate. The negative predictive value for nodal restaging is high (up to 95%), which is in part due to the high chance of sterilization.[19] An optimal size cutoff is lacking, but for practical

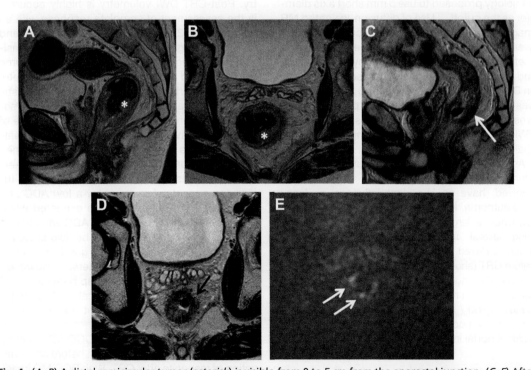

Fig. 4. (*A, B*) A distal semicircular tumor (*asterisk*) is visible from 0 to 5 cm from the anorectal junction. (*C–E*) After CRT, a residual wall thickening with heterogeneous signal with perirectal stranding is visible (*arrows*). Based on T2-weighted imaging, this is suspicious for a residual tumor, which is confirmed by the diffusion restriction in E. After surgery, the patient had a ypT3abN0 tumor.

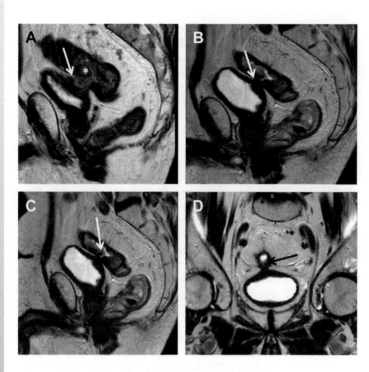

Fig. 5. A high rectosigmoidal tumor (*asterisk*) is shown with invasion into the bladder (*A, arrow*). After CRT, there is evident downsizing and the area of bladder invasion has become fibrotic (*B, arrow*). On the luminal side (*C, D, arrow*), there is still residual tumor in the rectosigmoid, which does not seem to extend into the bladder wall. However, it is not possible based on MR imaging to exclude the presence of small residual tumor islets in this fibrosis, so the surgeon needs to remove the fibrosis and thus a part of the bladder wall.

purposes a consensus guideline from the European Society of Gastrointestinal and Abdominal Radiology proposed to use 5 mm short axis diameter as the cutoff.[20] Use of diffusion-weighted MR imaging is not useful for the discrimination between benign and malignant nodes, but can be useful to detect nodes. An article by van Heeswijk and colleagues[21] showed that absence of nodes on DWI after CRT is a sign of ypN0, but this study was underpowered with only 10 patients (11%) presenting with absence of nodes after CRT on DWI. For now, nodal restaging remains a challenge.

An important separate nodal category are the lateral nodes, because these nodes, when involved, have an important influence on long-term outcome. Kusters and colleagues[22] recently published a large multi-institutional study evaluating lateral nodes before and after CRT, which showed that nodes 7 mm or greater before CRT (short axis) were likely to be malignant. Specifically, nodes in the internal iliac nodes showed a high risk for local recurrence.[22]

Figs. 6 and **7** show examples of nodal response with evident nodal sterilization, but also a case of residual nodal involvement after CRT.

QUANTITATIVE IMAGING

Several studies have evaluated quantitative and functional MR imaging during the last years to assess response to CRT. One of the easiest ways to quantitatively assess DWI is by volumetry. Post-CRT DWI volumetry is highly accurate in the assessment of complete response with an accuracy of 92% for post-CRT DWI volume and 86% for change in volume on DWI.[23] The sensitivity and specificity for post-CRT DWI volume were 70% and 98%, respectively. DWI volumetry clearly outperformed T2W volumetry. Mostly studied is quantitative assessment of DWI sequences, where the before, after, and change of ADC value have been evaluated. The pretreatment ADC has been reported to be higher when patients responds poorly to CRT, which is likely due to the presence of necrosis or mucinous tumor components. Tumors show a low ADC and an increase in ADC is therefore expected when response occurs. The post-CRT ADC and change in ADC have been shown to be (significantly) higher in patients with a good response compared with poor responders.[24] However, ADC values tend to show overlap between good and poor responders, which makes ADC measurements less useful in current routine clinical practice.

Dynamic contrast-enhanced (DCE) MR imaging has been evaluated for prediction before and evaluation of response after CRT. With DCE-MR imaging the tissue perfusion is studied and can be assessed quantitatively (measurement of K_{trans}, a measure of vessel permeability, K_{ep}, the flow rate

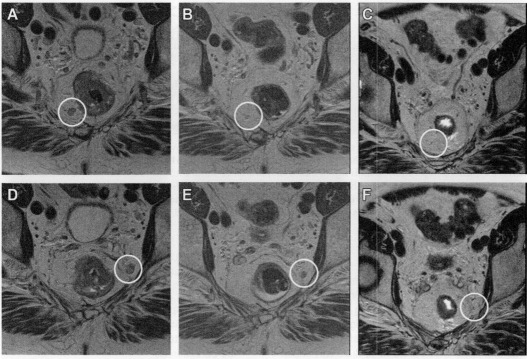

Fig. 6. (*A–C*) A mesorectal suspicious node (*circles*) is shown (*A*) before CRT, (*B*) after CRT, and (*C*) after long term follow-up during a wait-and-see policy. (*D–F*) A suspicious lateral node (circles) in the same patient (*D*) before CRT, (*E*) after CRT and (*F*) during follow-up. Both nodes show ongoing size decrease and only have a short axis of approximately 1 to 2 mm during long-term follow-up.

constant and V_e, the extracellular volume of fluid) or semiquantitatively (by assessing the signal-time-intensity curve). Several studies have reported that a high pre-CRT K_{trans} and a large decrease in K_{trans} after CRT are associated with good and/or complete response.[25] Semiquantitative DCE analyses were only sparsely studied. However, in current clinical practice DCE-MR imaging does not play a role in rectal cancer restaging.

Some other techniques have been studied like magnetic transfer imaging, BOLD imaging (blood oxygenation level-dependent imaging) and advanced diffusion analyses, based on intravoxel incoherent motion to assess the perfusion fraction.[24] These techniques, however, are only used in research settings and only preliminary results have been reported.

Radiomics has been introduced during the last years and has been studied within rectal cancer.[26,27] Radiomics make use of acquired data, but by applying advanced postprocessing methods more information can be captured than visible with the naked eye. Radiomics have shown promise, but needs to be extensively validated before steps toward clinical implementation can be taken.

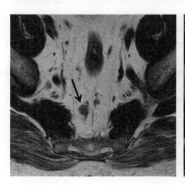
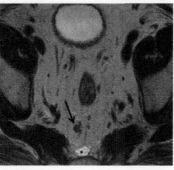

Fig. 7. On the left, a suspicious node (*arrow*; round enlarged [8 mm short axis] irregular node) is shown before CRT. After CRT on the right, there is downsizing, but the node (*arrow*) still has a short axis diameter of 6 mm and is round and irregular. Therefore, this node is still suspicious for malignancy, which was confirmed at histopathology after resection. Note the fluid presacrally (*asterisk*), which sometimes occurs after CRT.

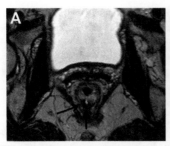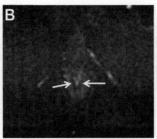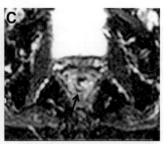

Fig. 8. (*A*) A post-CRT image is shown of a tumor that has responded very well with only minor fibrotic mucosal signal change from 5 to 8 o'clock (*black arrows*). (*B*) The corresponding b1000 diffusion images are shown, in which the typical configuration of high signal based on luminal T2 shine through is visible (between the *arrows*), which does not correspond with the fibrosis that is visible on T2W MR imaging and is thus not residual tumor. (*C*) The ADC map is shown in which T2 dark through is seen at the location of the fibrosis (*black arrow*), owing to the high collagen content in fibrosis. This is not accompanied by high signal on diffusion and is thus not suspicious for residual tumor.

PITFALLS

Main pitfalls are applicable to DWI after CRT. One important pitfall is incorrect interpretation of T2 shine through. Tissues with a long T2 relaxation time can be can remain bright on high b-value images, owing to the T2-weighted nature of a DWI sequence. After CRT intraluminal fluid can cause T2 shine through, which can be mistaken for rectal wall diffusion abnormalities. In these cases, correlation with the ADC map is necessary to distinguish between T2 shine through (high ADC) and diffusion restriction (low ADC). Additionally, high signal on diffusion in a U-shape or star-shape is almost always intraluminal (**Fig. 8**). Mucinous tumors will show T2 shin- through as well, which makes DWI less useful for evaluation of mucinous tumors.

A second pitfall is T2 dark through (see **Fig. 8**), which refers to the low signal that is sometimes visible on the ADC map in fibrotic areas.[24] The high amount of collagen leads to this low signal and so it does not correspond with residual tumor. It is important to always compare the ADC with the high b-value DW images, as in cases of fibrosis no high signal on DWI will be seen, although in residual tumor there will be high signal on the high b-value images.

Artifacts (susceptibility owing to air) can cause high signal on the DW images and this can hamper image interpretation. Specifically smaller artifacts can be difficult to identify and might be mistaken for tumor. Use of an enema before the examination has been shown to decrease susceptibility artifacts.[28]

WHAT THE REFERRING PHYSICIAN NEEDS TO KNOW

The radiologist plays an important role in the restaging of rectal cancer, because the MR imaging will guide treatment decision making. The referring physician (mostly a surgeon) will need to know:

- Is there response or progression?
- In case of good response: can the response be complete and thus a wait-and-see policy be considered?
- What is the extent of residual tumor (tumor height, ycT stage and relation with surrounding structures)?
- Whether there are any findings that threaten a complete resection (eg, residual MRF invasion, sphincter invasion or ycT4 tumor)
- Response of nodes (including lateral nodes)

To capture these items, it is recommendable to use a structured report or checklist when reporting post-CRT MR imaging in rectal cancer.

SUMMARY

MR imaging plays a crucial role in post-CRT assessment of rectal cancer. Radiologists should assess response or progression, the possibility of a complete response, risk factors for incomplete resection, and nodal stage. Combining T2W MR imaging with DWI yields the best results to identify a complete response with MR imaging, but endoscopy is also of major importance. Overstaging of transmural invasion and MRF invasion after CRT occur regularly, owing to residual stranding that will be regarded as tumor to err on the safe side. Nodal restaging is a challenge. A structured report format or checklist is recommended when evaluating post-CRT MR imaging in rectal cancer.

REFERENCES

1. Collette L, Bosset J-F, Dulk Md, et al. Patients with curative resection of cT3-4 rectal cancer after

preoperative radiotherapy or radiochemotherapy: does anybody benefit from adjuvant fluorouracil-based chemotherapy? a trial of the European Organisation for Research and Treatment of Cancer Radiation Oncology Group. J Clin Oncol 2007;25(28): 4379–86.

2. Benson AB, Venook AP, Al-Hawary MM, et al. Rectal cancer, version 2.2018, NCCN clinical practice guidelines in oncology. J Natl Compr Canc Netw 2018;16(7):874.

3. Maas M, Nelemans PJ, Valentini V, et al. Long-term outcome in patients with a pathological complete response after chemoradiation for rectal cancer: a pooled analysis of individual patient data. Lancet Oncol 2010;11(9):835–44.

4. Heijnen LA, Maas M, Beets-Tan RG, et al. Nodal staging in rectal cancer: why is restaging after chemoradiation more accurate than primary nodal staging? Int J Colorectal Dis 2016;31(6):1157–62.

5. Maas M, Lambregts DM, Nelemans PJ, et al. Assessment of clinical complete response after chemoradiation for rectal cancer with digital rectal examination, endoscopy, and MRI: selection for organ-saving treatment. Ann Surg Oncol 2015; 22(12):3873–80.

6. Lambregts DMJ, Delli Pizzi A, Lahaye MJ, et al. A pattern-based approach combining tumor morphology on MRI with distinct signal patterns on diffusion-weighted imaging to assess response of rectal tumors after chemoradiotherapy. Dis Colon Rectum 2018;61(3):328–37.

7. van der Paardt MP, Zagers MB, Beets-Tan RG, et al. Patients who undergo preoperative chemoradiotherapy for locally advanced rectal cancer restaged by using diagnostic MR imaging: a systematic review and meta-analysis. Radiology 2013;269(1):101–12.

8. Patel UB, Brown G, Rutten H, et al. Comparison of magnetic resonance imaging and histopathological response to chemoradiotherapy in locally advanced rectal cancer. Ann Surg Oncol 2012;19(9):2842–52.

9. Mandard AM, Dalibard F, Mandard JC, et al. Pathologic assessment of tumor regression after preoperative chemoradiotherapy of esophageal carcinoma. Cancer 1994;73(11):2680–6.

10. Sclafani F, Brown G, Cunningham D, et al. Comparison between MRI and pathology in the assessment of tumour regression grade in rectal cancer. Br J Cancer 2017;117(10):1478.

11. Lambregts DM, Vandecaveye V, Barbaro B, et al. Diffusion-weighted MRI for selection of complete responders after chemoradiation for locally advanced rectal cancer: a multicenter study. Ann Surg Oncol 2011;18(8):2224–31.

12. Habr-Gama A, Perez RO, Nadalin W, et al. Operative versus nonoperative treatment for stage 0 distal rectal cancer following chemoradiation therapy: long-term results. Ann Surg 2004;240(4):711.

13. Van Der Valk MJ, Hilling DE, Bastiaannet E, et al. Long-term outcomes of clinical complete responders after neoadjuvant treatment for rectal cancer in the International Watch & Wait Database (IWWD): an international multicentre registry study. Lancet 2018;391(10139):2537–45.

14. Maas M, Beets-Tan RG, Lambregts DM, et al. Wait-and-see policy for clinical complete responders after chemoradiation for rectal cancer. J Clin Oncol 2011;29(35):4633–40.

15. Kim DJ, Kim JH, Lim JS, et al. Restaging of rectal cancer with MR imaging after concurrent chemotherapy and radiation therapy. Radiographics 2010;30(2):503–16.

16. Dresen RC, Beets GL, Rutten HJ, et al. Locally advanced rectal cancer: MR imaging for restaging after neoadjuvant radiation therapy with concomitant chemotherapy. Part I. Are we able to predict tumor confined to the rectal wall? Radiology 2009;252(1): 71–80.

17. Krdzalic J, Maas M, Engelen S, et al. MRI can accurately predict sphincter preservation after chemoradiation [Abstract ECR 2017]. Insights Imaging 2017; 8(Suppl 1):187.

18. Wang C, Zhou Z-G, Wang Z, et al. Nodal spread and micrometastasis within mesorectum. World J Gastroenterol 2005;11(23):3586.

19. Lahaye MJ, Beets GL, Engelen SM, et al. Locally advanced rectal cancer: MR imaging for restaging after neoadjuvant radiation therapy with concomitant chemotherapy part II. What are the criteria to predict involved lymph nodes? Radiology 2009;252(1): 81–91.

20. Beets-Tan RG, Lambregts DM, Maas M, et al. Magnetic resonance imaging for clinical management of rectal cancer: updated recommendations from the 2016 European Society of Gastrointestinal and Abdominal Radiology (ESGAR) consensus meeting. Eur Radiol 2018;28(4):1465–75.

21. Van Heeswijk MM, Lambregts DM, Palm WM, et al. DWI for assessment of rectal cancer nodes after chemoradiotherapy: is the absence of nodes at DWI proof of a negative nodal status? AJR Am J Roentgenol 2017;208(3):W79–84.

22. Ogura A, Konishi T, Cunningham C, et al. Neoadjuvant (Chemo) radiotherapy with total Mesorectal excision only is not sufficient to prevent lateral local recurrence in enlarged nodes: results of the Multicenter lateral node study of patients with low cT3/4 rectal cancer. J Clin Oncol 2019;37(1):33.

23. Lambregts DM, Rao S-X, Sassen S, et al. MRI and Diffusion-weighted MRI volumetry for identification of complete tumor responders after preoperative chemoradiotherapy in patients with rectal cancer. Ann Surg 2015;262(6):1034–9.

24. Lambregts DM, Boellaard TN, Beets-Tan RGH. Response evaluation after neoadjuvant treatment

for rectal cancer using modern MR imaging: a pictorial review. Insights Imaging 2019;10(1):15.

25. Dijkhoff RA, Beets-Tan RG, Lambregts DM, et al. Value of DCE-MRI for staging and response evaluation in rectal cancer: a systematic review. Eur J Radiol 2017;95:155–68.

26. Bibault J-E, Giraud P, Durdux C, et al. Deep Learning and Radiomics predict complete response after neo-adjuvant chemoradiation for locally advanced rectal cancer. Sci Rep 2018;8(1):12611.

27. Cui Y, Yang X, Shi Z, et al. Radiomics analysis of multiparametric MRI for prediction of pathological complete response to neoadjuvant chemoradiotherapy in locally advanced rectal cancer. Eur Radiol 2019;29(3):1211–20.

28. van Griethuysen JJ, Bus EM, Hauptmann M, et al. Gas-induced susceptibility artefacts on diffusion-weighted MRI of the rectum at 1.5 T–Effect of applying a micro-enema to improve image quality. Eur J Radiol 2018;99:131–7.

Staging of Anal Cancer
Role of MR Imaging

Monique Maas, MD, PhD[a],*, Jeroen A.W. Tielbeek, MD, PhD[b], Jaap Stoker, MD, PhD[b]

KEYWORDS

- Anal cancer • MR imaging • Staging • Post-chemoradiation evaluation • Recurrence
- Differential diagnosis

KEY POINTS

- Anal cancer is a relatively rare malignancy and treatment mostly consists of chemoradiation.
- T staging depends on tumor size and on invasion of surrounding organs.
- N staging is determined by nodal location.
- MR imaging is the mainstay of local staging and is performed at primary staging and 6 to 8 weeks after chemoradiation therapy to assess tumor and nodal response.
- Maximal response is expected at 6 months from chemoradiation therapy, and a complete response is obtained in 90% of patients.

INTRODUCTION

Anal cancer is a relatively rare malignancy that occurs in the anal canal or the perianal skin within 5 cm of the anal margin. Approximately 8200 new cases are found annually in the United States and anal cancer makes up 2.6% of all digestive cancers.[1] The majority of cases concern squamous cell carcinoma; less common are adenocarcinoma or melanoma. Most patients present with anal itch, bleeding or pain. However, some patients are asymptomatic. Often complaints are mistaken for hemorrhoids or fissures, leading to a substantial delay in diagnosis in many cases. Risk factors for anal cancer are presence of human papillomavirus, human immunodeficiency virus seropositivity, smoking, passive anal intercourse, and having multiple sex partners.[2] Staging is performed by clinical examination with proctoscopy, ultrasound (inguinal area) examination, MR imaging, and 18F-fluorodesoxyglucose positron emission tomography computed tomography

(^{18}F-FDG PET-CT) scans. Treatment is aimed at providing cure while maintaining the best sphincter function possible. Depending on the location and staging, treatment can consist of surgery (local excision or abdominoperineal resection) and/or chemoradiation. Tumors in the anal margin (the skin surrounding the anal verge) are generally treated with local excision. Tumors in the anal canal itself are usually too large to excise locally (local excision is only an option in tumors <1 cm) and in these cases chemoradiation is given. Radiation preferably consists of intensity-modulated radiotherapy, to achieve the lowest toxicity possible. Chemoradiation consists of a total dose of 45.0 to 50.4 Gy on the primary target area, delivered in fractions of 1.8 to 2.0 Gy. This treatment is usually followed by a boost of radiation of 15 to 25 Gy.[3] The radiation field includes the primary tumor, the anal canal and margin and regional nodal areas (in tumors >1–2 cm or N+ stage). Regional nodal areas include the internal pudendal nodes, internal and external iliac

Disclosure Statement: J. Stoker is research consultant for Robarts Clinical Trials and has a research grant by Takeda; both not related to the topic of this article.
[a] Department of Radiology, The Netherlands Cancer Institute, PO Box 90203, Amsterdam 1006BE, the Netherlands; [b] Department of Radiology and Nuclear Medicine, Amsterdam UMC, Location AMC, University of Amsterdam, PO Box 22660, 1100DD Amsterdam Zuid-Oost, the Netherlands
* Corresponding author.
E-mail address: m.maas@nki.nl

Magn Reson Imaging Clin N Am 28 (2020) 127–140
https://doi.org/10.1016/j.mric.2019.09.005
1064-9689/20/© 2019 Elsevier Inc. All rights reserved.

mri.theclinics.com

nodes and the mesorectal nodes for tumors above the dentate line. For tumors below the dentate line, inguinal nodes are irradiated as well. Concomitant chemotherapy consists of mitomycin C combined with capecitabine or 5-fluorouracil or 5-fluorouracil with cisplatin. When there is N+ disease, there will generally be a boost on the involved nodal regions or lymph node dissection will be performed.[3]

Maximal response is obtained 6 months after chemoradiation.[4] In 80% to 90% of cases, a complete response is found and the patient is then followed up. In case of an incomplete response, salvage surgery can be performed by abdominoperineal resection, combined with groin dissection in case of metastatic inguinal nodes. Sometimes (if extensive invasion is present) it is necessary to perform a larger excision (by extralevatoric abdominoperineal resection). In case of recurrence, abdominoperineal resection is the treatment of choice, if possible.

NORMAL ANATOMY AND IMAGING TECHNIQUES
Anatomy

The anal anatomy comprises multiple cylindrical layers (**Fig. 1**). Innermost is the mucosa and submucosa lining the anal canal; in the inferior part this is (sub)epithelium. Next is the smooth muscle internal sphincter, which is the continuation of the circular layer of the rectal wall. The internal sphincter lower edge is approximately 1 cm above the caudal edge of the anal sphincter. Next is the intersphincteric space with next to this the outer striated muscle layer of the anal sphincter that constitutes the circular external sphincter and sling-like puborectal muscle. The external sphincter is approximately the lower half of the outer layer and the puborectal muscle

the upper outer half. The anal sphincter is continuous with the rectum at the anorectal junction, with at this level also the levator plate that attaches to the fascia of the internal obturator muscle.

Imaging Technique and Protocol

For local evaluation MR imaging is the main modality in anal cancer, specifically for tumors of 2 cm and larger. At least 90% of the cases the anal cancer is visible on MR imaging. MR imaging offers a high spatial resolution and can demonstrate anal anatomy most accurate. A typical protocol consists of 3 T2-weighted sequences in sagittal, axial and coronal plane, angled perpendicular or parallel to the anal canal. A T1-weighted sequence covering the whole pelvis is required to image nodal disease. A fat-saturated T2 sequence can be used in case of pre-existing fistulae. Additionally, a diffusion-weighted imaging (DWI) sequence can be used, which can help in identification of a lesion and has potential to help in response assessment after chemoradiation, similar to rectal cancer.

Whole body staging for locoregional nodes, distant nodes and distant metastases is performed with a ^{18}F-FDG-PET-CT scan. The area from groin to skull base is covered. Anal cancers are almost always highly ^{18}F-FDG avid and thus sensitivity for metastases is high.

For nodal staging of the groin area ultrasound with fine needle aspiration is used, sometimes routinely, but often after ^{18}F-FDG-PET-CT scan to perform aspiration based on suspicious nodes on ^{18}F-FDG-PET-CT scan. More distant nodes are staged with MR imaging and/or ^{18}F-FDG-PET-CT scan.

Endorectal ultrasound (EUS) is useful to evaluate local transmural extension of the tumor, but only in experienced hands. EUS is not valuable

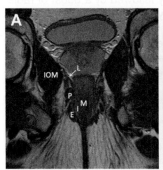 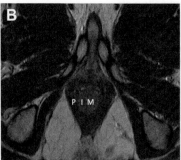 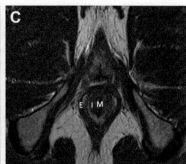

Fig. 1. The anal anatomy is shown in (*A*) a coronal T2W and (*B–C*) 2 axial T2W images. (*A–C*) The images show the mucosa/submucosa (M), the internal sphincter (I), and the outer striated muscle layer of the anal sphincter that constitutes the external sphincter (E) and puborectal muscle (P). (*A*) Image also shows the levator plate (L) that attaches to the fascia of the internal obturator muscle (IOM).

for nodal staging, therefore, MR imaging is the mainstay of imaging the local disease in anal cancer.[3,5]

IMAGING FINDINGS AND DIAGNOSTIC CRITERIA OF ANAL CANCER
T Stage

The T stage in anal cancer is based on tumor size. T1 tumors are up to 2 cm in size; T2 tumors 2 to 5 cm; T3 tumors larger than 5 cm; and when a tumor invades other structures it is a T4 tumor.[6] Structures that can be invaded and will classify the tumor as T4 are puborectal or levator muscle, prostate, seminal vesicles, vagina, uterus/adnexa, bone, piriform muscle, or obturator muscles. Specifically, direct invasion in the rectal wall, perineal skin, and perianal subcutaneous tissues and the internal and/or external sphincter muscle are not deemed as T4 tumors.[7] In tumors with T stage 2 to 4 chemoradiation is indicated; depending on the location in T1 tumors local excision or chemoradiation can both be considered.

T staging is performed by MR imaging primarily, but as briefly mentioned, there is also a role for EUS. EUS has been reported to be able to show the anal cancer in 100% of the cases.[8] Also, evaluation of T1 tumors EUS is a good option, mainly because MR imaging has difficulty to detect such small lesions. ^{18}F-FDG-PET-CT scans can detect almost all lesions (99% detection rate), but is not helpful for T staging.[9]

DWI can help in the detection of the anal cancer, when it is difficult to identify the tumor on T2-weighted images. For T staging DWI is not advised, but a recent article has shown that DWI-based volumetry of the tumor (to establish the target volume for radiation) leads to a lower size measurement of the tumor than if T2-weighted (T2W) MR imaging if used.[10] So, possibly DWI can have a role in tumor staging, but this needs to be explored.

N Stage

Once evaluation of the primary tumor has been completed, whole body imaging should be performed to evaluate for lymphadenopathy or distant metastasis. According to the eighth TNM staging edition, N stage can be categorized into 5 categories, depending on the location of the nodes, whereas in the seventh edition only the number of malignant nodes was relevant for N staging. The eighth TNM staging edition is based on the regional lymphatic drainage of the anorectal region.[6] Regional nodal metastasis spreads to the inguinal regions (mostly in tumors confined to the anal canal below the dentate line), mesorectal compartment (if above the dentate line or when the rectal wall is involved), and/or the internal and external iliac chain. In the nodal staging classification system, N0 means that there are no regional lymph node metastases. N1 indicates regional lymph node metastases and is divided into 3 categories: N1a, metastasis in inguinal, mesorectal and/or internal iliac nodes; N1b, metastasis in external iliac nodes; and N1c, metastasis in external iliac and in inguinal, mesorectal and/or internal iliac nodes (so, a combination of N1a and N1b). Nodes further along the common iliac artery or aorta are considered M1 disease. Nx indicates that nodal stage cannot be assessed or is not assessed yet. In about 25% to 45% of anal cancers, there is nodal involvement.[11] Nodal involvement leads to a higher risk for local failure and a worse 5-year disease-free and overall survival in patients with T2 to T4 tumors.[12]

Locoregional nodes are depicted on MR imaging, but as in other cancers, it is challenging to stage nodes based on anatomic imaging such as MR imaging and CT scanning. Size criteria often lead to substantial understaging and overstaging. Therefore, nodal staging relies on ultrasound and ^{18}F-FDG-PET-CT scans. Ultrasound signs of malignancy are round shape, short axis size of greater than 1 cm, loss of fatty hilum, and a thickened or asymmetric cortex. Usually in stage cT1 and greater anal cancer ^{18}F-FDG-PET-CT scanning is performed and nodal spread can be evaluated. Based on the results of the ^{18}F-FDG-PET-CT scan, targeted ultrasound imaging can be performed to evaluate the morphologic aspect and size of inguinal nodes and perform a fine needle aspiration in ^{18}F-FDG avid or morphologically suspicious nodes. When nodes are evaluated on MR imaging and CT scans, enlargement and the presence of necrosis will be the most suspicious features for node malignancy. Additionally, irregularity, asymmetry, or signal heterogeneity are suspicious findings and these findings are best assessed by MR imaging given the high spatial resolution and high contrast between tissues. Unfortunately, size criteria have a disappointing accuracy (leading to false-negative findings in small nodes and false-positive findings in large nodes), similar to the accuracy in rectal cancer (with a sensitivity of 66% and specificity of 76%).[13] When using MR imaging for nodal staging, short axis size cutoffs of 8, 5, and 10 mm have been proposed for pelvic, mesorectal, and inguinal nodes, respectively.[14] These morphologic criteria are less easy to apply in nodes less than 5 mm. ^{18}F-FDG-PET-CT scanning provides better accuracy for nodal staging, with an alteration in nodal stage in 28% of the cases when added after other imaging.[9] A meta-analysis from Jones and colleagues[9] reported a sensitivity of 99% for nodal staging by ^{18}F-FDG-PET-CT scan, compared with 60% with a CT scan. However, another meta-analysis reported a pooled sensitivity of only 56% for ^{18}F-FDG-PET-CT scan.[15] Specificity is high and ranges from 90% to 100%, respectively.[9] However, ^{18}F-FDG-PET-CT scanning has a limited resolution and can miss metastases in nodes less than 5 mm. So, in current practice small nodes in particular pose a problem. **Figs. 2–6** show several examples of anal cancers with different T and N stages.

M Staging

As mentioned, nodes further along the common iliac artery or aorta are considered M1 disease. M staging is only based on the absence or presence of metastases. In the TNM classification M0 means no distant metastasis and M1 means distant metastasis. For anal cancer, no difference is made between regional, solitary or multiple metastases. The literature shows that approximately 6% of squamous cell anal carcinomas are metastatic at diagnosis.[16,17] Patients with metastatic disease have a prognosis with 5-year median overall survival rates of 10% in men and 20% in women.[18]

A particular group easily overlooked is nodes just below the aortic bifurcation. Beside the lymph nodes, mainly the liver and the lungs are involved.

To rule out distant metastases, a chest and abdomen CT scan with intravenous contrast is advised. Preparation with oral contrast is advised in the National Comprehensive Cancer Network 2017 guidelines, but preparation with water is sufficient in the authors' experiences.[3] If available, ^{18}F-FDG-PET-CT scanning can be considered. Anal cancers and their metastases are almost always highly FGD avid and sensitivity for metastases is therefore high. A systemic review proposes that ^{18}F-FDG-PET-CT scans may aid in treatment monitoring and might help in the selection of patients who may benefit from more aggressive treatment.[19] Therefore, ^{18}F-FDG-PET-CT scans might be helpful for monitoring therapy, the detection of recurrent disease and establishing the presence of distant metastases.[20] However, the National Comprehensive Cancer Network 2017 guidelines do not consider ^{18}F-FDG-PET-CT scans to be a replacement for a diagnostic CT scan.[3]

EVALUATION AFTER CHEMORADIATION THERAPY

Postchemoradiation evaluation with MR imaging is usually performed approximately 6 to 10 weeks after the last radiation dose. At this point, there is usually a good response, but, because maximal response can take up to 6 months to occur, usually residual tumor is still present. For this reason, MR imaging was already deemed unhelpful for postchemoradiation evaluation of anal cancer in 2010 by Goh and colleagues.[21] Despite this study, MR imaging is still used after chemoradiation to

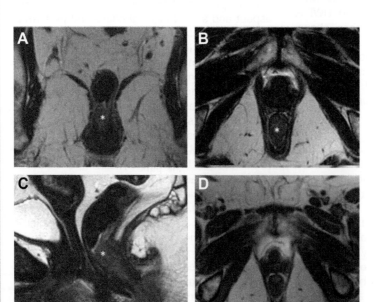

Fig. 2. (A) Coronal T2W image shows an anal cancer of 2.2 cm (*asterisk*) confined to the anal canal. (B) Images show the axial plane and (C) the sagittal plane. (D) Image shows the inguinal areas without suspicious nodes. This patient has a cT2N0 tumor.

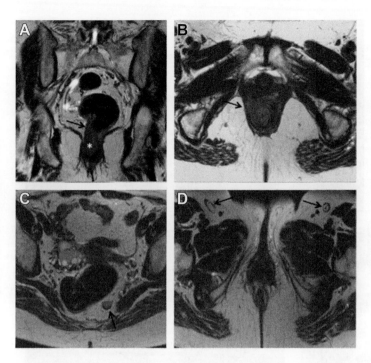

Fig. 3. (A) Coronal T2W image shows an anal cancer of 5.3 cm (*asterisk*) with rectal invasion (*black arrow*). (B) The axial plane with extension through the m. puborectalis (*black arrow*). (C) A malignant mesorectal node is seen (*black arrow*). (D) Image shows typically normal benign inguinal nodes in the same patient (*black arrows*). This patient has a cT3N1a tumor.

confirm that there is response and to describe what the size and extension of the (residual) tumor are as a baseline for later follow-up. At this timepoint, the initial response is assessed and nodes can be reevaluated. To detect a complete response MR imaging would have to be performed later (at 6 months), but response evaluation at 6 months and during follow-up is done by clinical

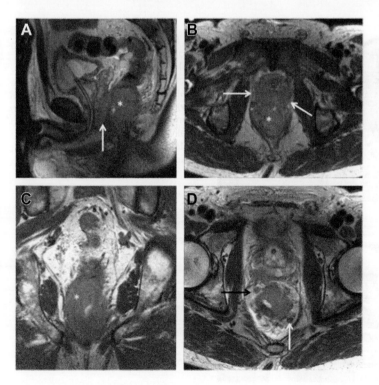

Fig. 4. (A) Sagittal T2W image shows an anal cancer (*asterisk*) that shows invasion into the prostate (*white arrows* in A and B). (B) The axial plane with extension through the puborectalis into the prostate. (C) The coronal plane with left levator plate invasion. (D) Multiple suspicious mesorectal nodes (*arrows*). This patient has a cT4N1a tumor.

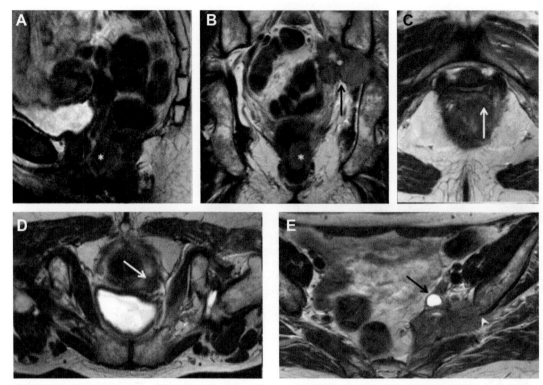

Fig. 5. (*A*) Sagittal T2W image with motion artifacts shows an anal tumor of 3.8 cm (*asterisk*). (*B*) A coronal image shows the tumor (*asterisk*) but also a large para-iliac tumor (*black arrow*). (*C*) Image shows posterior vaginal wall invasion (*white arrow*) and (*D*) another image shows a deposit in the mesorectal fascia (*white arrow*). (*E*) A dilated ureter (*black arrow*) is visible owing to obstruction by the para-iliac mass (probably node metastasis). Note the bone invasion (white *arrowhead*). This patient has a cT4N1a tumor.

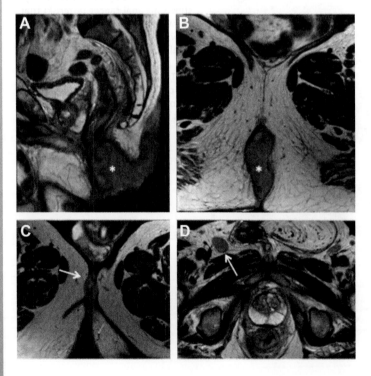

Fig. 6. (*A*) Sagittal T2W image and (*B*) a coronal T2W image shows a large anal cancer of 7 cm (*asterisk*) with extensive growth caudally. (*C*) In the axial view, a second nodule (*white arrow*) is found perineally (separate from the anal tumor). (*D*) Another axial view shows a malignant inguinal node on the right (*white arrow*). This patient has a cT3N1a tumor.

examination. Follow-up consists of 3 to 6 monthly clinical examinations and MR imaging will only be performed when there is a suspected recurrence or if there is persistent residual tumor clinically after 6 months. Then, staging of the residual tumor will be performed according to the same TNM stages as described for primary staging.

Anal tumors respond to chemoradiation by fibrotic change. Just as for rectal cancer, fibrosis is hypointense at T2W MR imaging and it is not possible to exclude the presence of small residual tumor islets in the fibrosis based on visual evaluation. Residual tumor shows the same characteristics on MR imaging as at primary staging. When evaluating postchemoradiation MR imaging for anal cancer, the same issues are evaluated as described during primary staging. Usually there is a size and signal intensity decrease, leading to a change in T stage. The decrease in size and signal intensity are concordant and most profound in complete responders.[14,22] **Fig. 7** shows an example of an anal tumor that had a complete response to chemoradiation. Addition of a contrast-enhanced T1-weighted sequence does not help in staging of anal cancer. Koh and colleagues[22] described long-term MR imaging features and reported that when signal intensity stabilizes 1 year after chemoradiation, this is suggestive of prolonged complete response. Kochhar and colleagues[23] have evaluated the tumor regression grade, as used in rectal cancer, for anal cancer response assessment. MR imaging was performed at 3 and 6 months after chemoradiation. In 74 patients, they found a tumor size reduction in 29% at 3 months and 81% at 6 months. Signal intensity decreased in up to 84% at 6 months. 92% had sterilization of primarily suspicious nodes. None of the patients with tumor regression grade 1 or 2 at 6 months developed local relapse. Agreement was moderate (0.61 and 0.76 at 3 and 6 months, respectively). They introduced the tram track sign as a potential predictor of complete response. The tram track sign is defined as occurrence of low signal bands between the inner and outer margin of the internal sphincter at the former tumor location. Of the 39 patients that showed the tram track sign, one developed a local relapse. However, this sign was only encountered in 57% of the patients at 6 months.[23] Also, given the postchemoradiation evaluation after 8 weeks rather than 6 months in current clinical practice, the clinical value of the tram track sign in current clinical practice is probably low.

One of the pitfalls on MR imaging is high signal edema in the mucosa owing to chemoradiation, which can lead to a pseudotumor appearance. This is particularly challenging because it is accompanied by focal thickening and because anal cancer generally shows high signal on T2.

After chemoradiation, DWI can be of help to discriminate a complete response from residual tumor, similar to rectal cancer. However, DWI for anal cancer has not yet been evaluated and is thus not routinely recommended. One study by

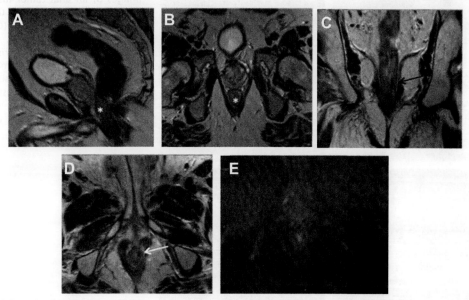

Fig. 7. (*A*) Sagittal and (*B*) axial T2W images show a T2 tumor of 2.5 cm (*asterisk*). (*C–E*) After chemoradiation, T2W images show only a small thin line of fibrosis (*black and white arrows*) at the former tumor location, (*E*) without diffusion restriction. This patient had a complete response and did not develop a recurrence.

Reginelli and colleagues[8] showed that in complete responders significantly less diffusion restriction is found than in residual tumors. However, postchemoradiation DWI in the anal canal can be challenging owing to postradiation effects, leading to high signal on high b-value DWI in complete responders, not corresponding with true residual tumor.

RECURRENT ANAL CANCER

Recurrent disease is defined as initial complete response to therapy, with subsequent positive biopsies, more than 6 months after the completion of chemoradiation. Up to 30% of patients with squamous cell carcinoma of the anal canal will fail treatment, with either persistent or locally recurrent disease.[24] Fifty percent of anal cancer recurrences occur within the first 2 years after treatment and are located around the primary site of disease or as lymph node metastases in the perirectal, presacral, and internal iliac chains.[14] Tumors that are likely to relapse are basaloid subtypes and patients after incomplete chemoradiation, with higher disease state or human immunodeficiency virus-positive status.[20,24,25] Follow-up imaging is important for assuring stability of appearance after treatment and for the detection of relapse. Early detection and accurate staging is essential because patients with disease relapse may benefit from more aggressive salvage surgery.

The high-contrast resolution of MR imaging makes it suitable for assessment of locoregional recurrence. Therefore, MR imaging is the preferred follow-up imaging modality in anal cancer and may assist in the early detection of recurrence. However, there is scarce literature on follow-up imaging of recurrences in anal cancer. Careful comparison with the initial post-treatment baseline MR imaging is crucial for early diagnosis of recurrence. After treatment, the same staging parameters are used as with baseline MR imaging scan. Recurrence is often seen as a new nodule or a mass isointense to the original tumor. **Fig. 8** shows an example of recurrent anal cancer after chemoradiation. As mentioned elsewhere in this article, whole body staging using CT or ^{18}F-FDG-PET-CT scanning is advised to rule out distant metastases.

DIFFERENTIAL DIAGNOSES AND PITFALLS

The differential diagnoses of anal carcinoma include several diseases, and most of these are rare. Here several important differential diagnoses are described.

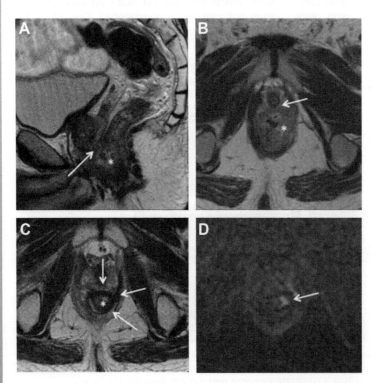

Fig. 8. (*A*) Sagittal and (*B*) axial T2W images show prechemoradiation images of an anal tumor (*asterisk*) that invades the posterior urethra and prostate (cT4; *arrows*). (*C*) During follow-up after 1 year, a new hyperintense mass (*asterisk*) is visible on the axial T2W image in the irradiated area (fibrosis indicated by *arrows*). (*D*) Diffusion restriction in the area is shown (*arrow*). This is consistent with a recurrence.

Gastrointestinal Stroma Cell Tumor

Gastrointestinal stroma cell tumors (GISTs) are assumed to originate from the interstitial cells of Cajal stem cells within the wall of the gastrointestinal tract. However, there is debate concerning this assumed origin given that GISTs arise in the omentum and mesenterium.

GISTs are the most common non-epithelial tumors of the gastrointestinal tract, but in fact are relatively rare (approximately 1% of primary gastrointestinal cancers). GISTs can occur anywhere in the gastrointestinal tract. However, the anus is a rare location for GIST; less than 1% of GISTs are reported to originate from the anal canal.[26] Rectal GIST can extend into the anal canal and—because GIST are often large tumors—it may be difficult to differentiate between anal or rectal origin. As at other locations in the gastrointestinal tract, GIST tumors are well-defined masses and especially large GISTs can be heterogeneous (**Fig. 9**).[27]

Anal Lymphoma

Anal lymphoma is very rare. It presents as a solid mass that is often isointense on non-enhanced T1-weighted MR sequences, shows intermediate enhancement and is hyperintense on T2-weighted sequences. It may present as a perianal abscess and might be misdiagnosed as such initially.[28] Gastrointestinal lymphoma is associated with autoimmune disorders, inflammatory bowel disease, immune deficiency, immune suppression, and advanced age (**Fig. 10**).

Rhabdomyosarcoma

Rhabdomyosarcoma originating from the anus and perianal region is very rare; the anus can also be involved in rhabdomyosarcomas extending into the anal region (**Fig. 11**).

Rhabdomyosarcoma present as soft tissue masses with intermediate signal intensity on T2-weighted sequences and extend into the surrounding structures and organs. In the differential diagnosis of anal carcinoma, there are important differences between these diseases. Differences include age at presentation, with rhabdomyosarcoma being a tumor basically presenting in childhood and adolescence. Further, rhabdomyosarcoma is often large at presentation and the histopathology is clearly different to anal carcinoma.

Aggressive Angiomyxomas

Aggressive angiomyxomas are mesenchymal tumors in the deep soft tissues that present as often large painless mass or cause local pressure effect. A laminated appearance, strong enhancement at MR imaging (contrary to CT scan), large vessels within the tumor and multicompartimental extension without involvement of other organs have been indicated as imaging features of aggressive angiomyxomas.[29] Sometimes cystic areas can be present. However, there are no pathognomonic features (**Fig. 12**).

Malignant Transformation of Perianal Fistulas

Perianal fistulas are easily differentiated from anal cancer based on clinical history and findings. However, in patients with long-standing perianal fistulas in Crohn's disease, the differential diagnosis can become more difficult, especially because these patients have a risk for malignant transformation. This malignant transformation to adenocarcinoma or squamous cell carcinoma can be difficult to detect clinically and might only be detected when the malignancy has spread extensively. Consecutive MR imaging examinations performed for monitoring

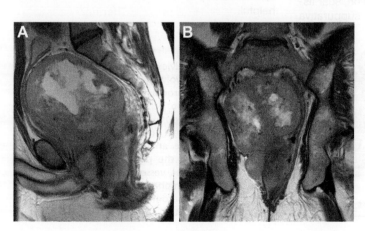

Fig. 9. (*A*) Sagittal and (*B*) coronal T2W turbo spin echo images show a large, smoothly demarcated, heterogeneous rectal GIST invading the anus in a male patient referred for feeling a mass, rectal blood loss, and dysuria.

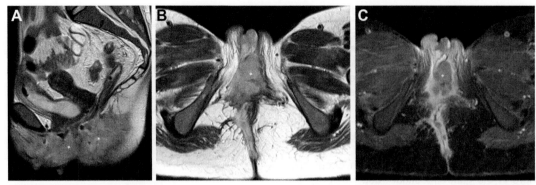

Fig. 10. (*A*) Sagittal and (*B*) axial T2W images show a large lymphoma (*asterisk*) in a female patient with long-standing Crohn's disease. (*C*) Axial T1W postcontrast image confirms the presence of a lymphoid mass (*asterisk*).

treatment of fistulous diseases can be instrumental in identifying malignant transformation, but malignancy can be hard to detect. One should scrutinize the sequences for suspicious features. These features include changes in signal intensity and the development of a soft tissue mass (**Fig. 13**). Active perianal fistulas have a T2 hyperintense core (inflammatory tissue and/or fluid) and surrounding hypo intense fibrous tissue; an inactive track will only show hypointense fibrous tissue. A malignancy will often present with intermediate signal intensity at T2-weighted imaging. At a contrast enhanced T1-weighted sequence inflammatory tissue will enhance intensively while fibrous tissue will show no or minimal enhancement; a malignancy will show intermediate signal intensity. At DWI the inflammatory core of the track or fistulous complex may show diffusion restriction whereas a malignancy shows diffuse diffusion restriction.

Hidradenitis Suppurativa

Hidradenitis suppurativa is a chronic inflammation of the process involving the skin and subcutaneous tissue resulting in abscess formation, scar tissue, and sinus tracks. Hidradenitis suppurativa

occurs primarily in intertriginous areas, including the inguinal area, perineum and perianal areas, buttocks, and gluteal cleft. The clinical manifestations of hidradenitis suppurativa are thought to be caused by follicular occlusion, follicular rupture, and an associated immune response. The usual onset of hidradenitis suppurativa is in the second or third decades of life, with women being more likely to develop this disease. Several factors influence the development of hidradenitis suppurativa, including genetic factors, mechanical stress, obesity, smoking, diet, and hormonal factors.

Based on the differences in presentation, clinically there will be rarely difficulty in differentiating between hidradenitis suppurativa and anal carcinoma. At MR imaging, contrary to anal carcinoma presenting as a mass, hidradenitis suppurativa presents with skin involvement, abscesses, tracks, and scarring (**Fig. 14**). In the setting of extensive disease with scarring and tracks extending to the anus, the differentiation might be less straightforward. Here the predominant location at the skin, lack of a soft tissue mass, together with clinical history and clinical findings will be very helpful.

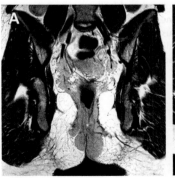
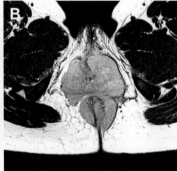

Fig. 11. A female patient with pelvic rhabdomyosarcoma, primarily involving the anal sphincter. (*A*) Coronal and (*B*) axial T2W turbo spin echo show a large homogeneous infiltrating rhabdomyosarcoma (*asterisk*) originating from the anal sphincter and extending to the pelvic floor and along the iliac vessels and to the perineum. Lymphadenopathy is visible. Some anatomic structures remain visible within the mass.

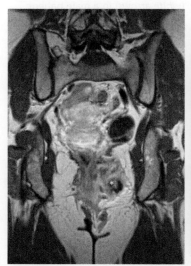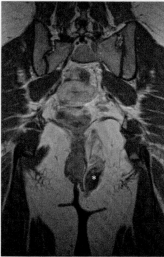

Fig. 12. Two coronal T2W images of an aggressive angiomyxoma (*asterisk*) in a female patient.

Anal Fissure

Primary anal fissures are caused by a tear of the superficial anal (sub)mucosa/(sub)epithelium (mostly posterior midline) by local trauma. Increased anal pressure in constipated patients is thought to be a major cause of anal fissure.

The posterior midline of the anal sphincter is the less perfused part of the anal sphincter. The tear of the anal (sub)mucosa/(sub)epithelium exposes the internal sphincter, which leads to spasms with pain and further decreased perfusion at the posterior midline.

Primary anal fissure should be differentiated from hemorrhoids (this can be difficult) and from anal fissures caused by other diseases—secondary anal fissures—such as in Crohn's disease, sarcoidosis, chlamydia, and in malignancy such as squamous cell anal cancer and leukemia. These secondary fissures can occur anywhere in the anus, in contrast with the mostly posterior midline position in primary anal fissures. The different clinical history and location are important in differential diagnoses.

At MR imaging anal fissure can be relatively subtle, as defects in the posterior midline (sub)mucosa/(sub)epithelium with some hyper intensity on T2-weighted sequences and enhancement on T1-weighted sequences (**Fig. 15**). Differentiation from hemorrhoids is often straightforward. Hemorrhoids commonly present as either luminal (or external) structures having the signal intensity of nearby vessels and a thin wall (except in case of thrombosis) (**Fig. 16**).

Anal Lipoma

The differentiation between anal carcinoma and anal lipoma often will be clinically manifest, but MR imaging might be helpful in this distinction, demonstrating the typical findings of a lipoma (**Fig. 17**).

This list of differential diagnoses for anal squamous call cancer is not conclusive. Several other diseases such as infectious diseases, lymphangioma, myofibroma, leiomyoma, leukemia, melanoma (**Fig. 18**), intraepithelial adenocarcinoma

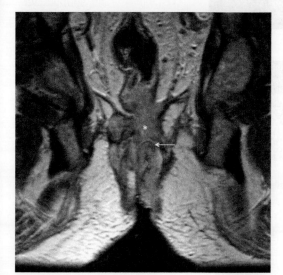

Fig. 13. A coronal T2W image shows the development of a malignant mass (*asterisk*) in a longstanding perianal fistula in a male patient with longstanding perianal Crohn's disease. A seton in one of the fistulas is still in situ (*white arrow*).

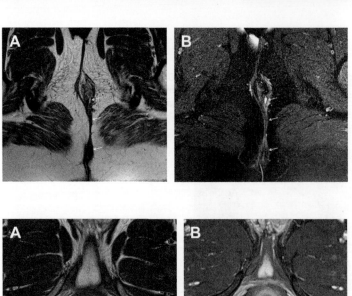

Fig. 14. Axial T2W images without (*A*) and with fat saturation (*B*) show hidradenitis suppurativa (*white arrows*) in a male patient.

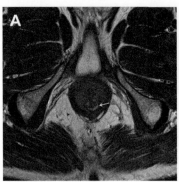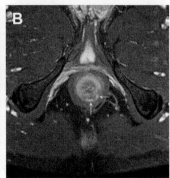

Fig. 15. (*A*) Axial T2W and (*B*) T1W postcontrast images in an human immunodeficiency virus positive patient with a deep anal fissure (*white arrows*); no malignancy at histopathology.

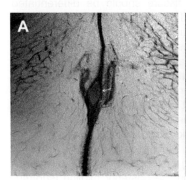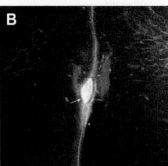

Fig. 16. (*A*) Axial oblique T2W and (*B*) fat-saturated T2W TSE image shows a hemorrhoid (*white arrows*) extending externally.

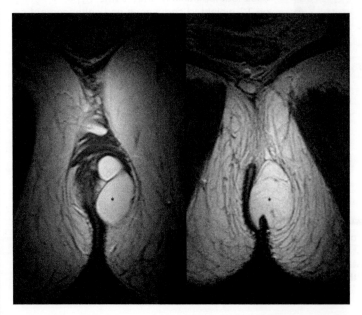

Fig. 17. A male patient with a swelling at the nates. Coronal T2-weighted turbo spin echo shows an anal lipoma (*asterisk*). In addition, there was a low signal intensity on fat saturated T2-weighted turbo spin echo images (not shown).

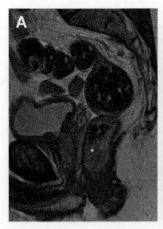 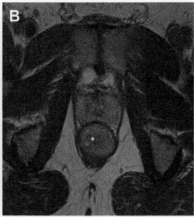

Fig. 18. (*A*) Sagittal and (*B*) axial T2W images show a round polypoid lesion at the anorectal junction (*asterisk*), with relatively hyperintense signal. The lesion is confined to the anorectal wall. This was a histologically proven anorectal melanoma. Patient was treated with transanal excision.

and verrucous carcinoma can be considered as well.[30]

SUMMARY: WHAT THE REFERRING PHYSICIAN NEEDS TO KNOW

Anal cancer is a rare malignancy. For local staging MR imaging is the mainstay to determine T stage, except for cT1 tumors, where EUS is more accurate than MR imaging. Anal cancer shows high signal on T2W-MR imaging and can be identified by DWI. T staging is based on lesion size or invasion into surrounding structures. Nodal staging is based on the location of nodes (mesorectal, iliac chain, inguinal). ^{18}F-FDG-PET-CT scanning is part of the staging procedure and is helpful for nodal staging and distant staging. EUS with fine needle aspiration is used for nodal staging in the inguinal area. Most anal cancers are treated with chemoradiation, which leads to a complete response in 80% to 90%. Surgery is indicated for small tumors and tumors in the anal margin or for noncomplete responders or locally recurrent disease. After chemoradiation tumor size and signal decrease and fibrosis occurs. Response evaluation is done by MR imaging at 6 to 10 weeks after chemoradiation, but maximal response is expected at 6 months. Therefore, the postchemoradiation MR imaging at 6 to 10 weeks is mostly used to assess initial response and reevaluate the nodes. Postradiation effects can hamper postchemoradiation evaluation and sometimes lead to overestimating residual tumor (eg, owing to edema). For locally recurrent disease, MR imaging and ^{18}F-FDG-PET-CT scans are used to evaluate the tumor extent and presence of metastases to and determine the treatment strategy. Follow-up to detect metastatic disease can be performed with CT scans with intravenous contrast, if

available ^{18}F-FDG-PET-CT scans can be considered. Metastatic anal cancer has a poor prognosis. When evaluating the anal canal, beware of the occurrence of anal cancer in perianal fistula. Also, many other entities can be found to mimic or obscure anal cancer; however, most are very rare. In these cases, MR imaging can be helpful to differentiate lesions.

REFERENCES

1. Siegel RL, Miller KD, Jemal A. Cancer statistics, 2017. CA Cancer J Clin 2017;67(1):7–30.
2. Moureau-Zabotto L, Vendrely V, Abramowitz L, et al. Anal cancer: French Intergroup clinical practice guidelines for diagnosis, treatment and follow-up (SNFGE, FFCD, GERCOR, UNICANCER, SFCD, SFED, SFRO, SNFCP). Dig Liver Dis 2017;49(8):831–40.
3. Al BB, Alan PV, Mahmoud MA-H, et al. Anal carcinoma, version 2.2018, NCCN clinical practice guidelines in oncology. J Natl Compr Canc Netw 2018;16(7):852–71.
4. Glynne-Jones R, Adams R, Lopes A, et al. Clinical endpoints in trials of chemoradiation for patients with anal cancer. Lancet Oncol 2017;18(4):e218–27.
5. Otto SD, Lee L, Buhr HJ, et al. Staging anal cancer: prospective comparison of transanal endoscopic ultrasound and magnetic resonance imaging. J Gastrointest Surg 2009;13(7):1292–8.
6. Brierley JD, Gospodarowicz MK, Wittekind C. TNM classification of malignant tumours. Hoboken (NJ): John Wiley & Sons; 2016.
7. Durot C, Dohan A, Boudiaf M, et al. Cancer of the anal canal: diagnosis, staging and follow-up with MRI. Korean J Radiol 2017;18(6):946–56.
8. Reginelli A, Granata V, Fusco R, et al. Diagnostic performance of magnetic resonance imaging and 3D endoanal ultrasound in detection, staging and

assessment post treatment, in anal cancer. Oncotarget 2017;8(14):22980–90.

9. Jones M, Hruby G, Solomon M, et al. The role of FDG-PET in the initial staging and response assessment of anal cancer: a systematic review and meta-analysis. Ann Surg Oncol 2015;22(11):3574–81.

10. Prezzi D, Mandegaran R, Gourtsoyianni S, et al. The impact of MRI sequence on tumour staging and gross tumour volume delineation in squamous cell carcinoma of the anal canal. Eur Radiol 2018; 28(4):1512–9.

11. Jederan E, Lovey J, Szentirmai Z, et al. The role of MRI in the assessment of the local status of anal carcinomas and in their management. Pathol Oncol Res 2015;21(3):571–9.

12. Gunderson LL, Moughan J, Ajani JA, et al. Anal carcinoma: impact of TN category of disease on survival, disease relapse, and colostomy failure in US Gastrointestinal Intergroup RTOG 98-11 phase 3 trial. Int J Radiat Oncol Biol Phys 2013;87(4):638–45.

13. Bipat S, Glas AS, Slors FJ, et al. Rectal cancer: local staging and assessment of lymph node involvement with endoluminal US, CT, and MR imaging–a meta-analysis. Radiology 2004;232(3):773–83.

14. Gourtsoyianni S, Goh V. MRI of anal cancer: assessing response to definitive chemoradiotherapy. Abdom Imaging 2014;39(1):2–17.

15. Caldarella C, Annunziata S, Treglia G, et al. Diagnostic performance of positron emission tomography/computed tomography using fluorine-18 fluorodeoxyglucose in detecting locoregional nodal involvement in patients with anal canal cancer: a systematic review and meta-analysis. ScientificWorldJournal 2014;2014:196068.

16. Bilimoria KY, Bentrem DJ, Rock CE, et al. Outcomes and prognostic factors for squamous-cell carcinoma of the anal canal: analysis of patients from the National Cancer Data Base. Dis Colon Rectum 2009; 52(4):624–31.

17. Abramowitz L, Mathieu N, Roudot-Thoraval F, et al. Epidermoid anal cancer prognosis comparison among HIV+ and HIV- patients. Aliment Pharmacol Ther 2009;30(4):414–21.

18. Johnson LG, Madeleine MM, Newcomer LM, et al. Anal cancer incidence and survival: the surveillance, epidemiology, and end results experience, 1973-2000. Cancer 2004;101(2):281–8.

19. Hong JC, Cui Y, Patel BN, et al. Association of interim FDG-PET imaging during chemoradiation for squamous anal canal carcinoma with recurrence. Int J Radiat Oncol Biol Phys 2018;102(4):1046–51.

20. Kochhar R, Plumb AA, Carrington BM, et al. Imaging of anal carcinoma. AJR Am J Roentgenol 2012; 199(3):W335–44.

21. Goh V, Gollub FK, Liaw J, et al. Magnetic resonance imaging assessment of squamous cell carcinoma of the anal canal before and after chemoradiation: can MRI predict for eventual clinical outcome? Int J Radiat Oncol Biol Phys 2010;78(3):715–21.

22. Koh DM, Dzik-Jurasz A, O'Neill B, et al. Pelvic phased-array MR imaging of anal carcinoma before and after chemoradiation. Br J Radiol 2008;81(962): 91–8.

23. Kochhar R, Renehan AG, Mullan D, et al. The assessment of local response using magnetic resonance imaging at 3- and 6-month post chemoradiotherapy in patients with anal cancer. Eur Radiol 2017;27(2):607–17.

24. Roohipour R, Patil S, Goodman KA, et al. Squamous-cell carcinoma of the anal canal: predictors of treatment outcome. Dis Colon Rectum 2008; 51(2):147–53.

25. Das P, Bhatia S, Eng C, et al. Predictors and patterns of recurrence after definitive chemoradiation for anal cancer. Int J Radiat Oncol Biol Phys 2007; 68(3):794–800.

26. Singhal S, Singhal A, Tugnait R, et al. Anorectal gastrointestinal stromal tumor: a case report and literature review. Case Rep Gastrointest Med 2013; 2013:934875.

27. Sandrasegaran K, Rajesh A, Rushing DA, et al. Gastrointestinal stromal tumors: CT and MRI findings. Eur Radiol 2005;15(7):1407–14.

28. Jayasekera H, Gorissen K, Francis L, et al. Diffuse large B cell lymphoma presenting as a peri-anal abscess. J Surg Case Rep 2014;2014(6) [pii:rju035].

29. Surabhi VR, Garg N, Frumovitz M, et al. Aggressive angiomyxomas: a comprehensive imaging review with clinical and histopathologic correlation. AJR Am J Roentgenol 2014;202(6):1171–8.

30. Surabhi VR, Menias CO, Amer AM, et al. Tumors and tumorlike conditions of the anal canal and perianal region: MR imaging findings. Radiographics 2016; 36(5):1339–53.

Magnetic Resonance Imaging of Fistula-In-Ano

Steve Halligan, MB BS, MD, PhD, FRCP, FRCR, FMedSci

KEYWORDS

• Anal fistula • Rectal fistula • Anus • Diseases • Magnetic resonance imaging • Anal gland

KEY POINTS

- Preoperative classification of fistula-in-ano is pivotal for successful surgical treatment because this determines what type of operation is performed.
- MR imaging is the most appropriate imaging modality with which to classify fistula-in-ano. It is more accurate than other imaging modalities and is even more accurate than examination under anesthetic overall.
- The major therapeutic impact of MR imaging lies with its ability to both identify the course of the fistula (thereby indicating the extent of any sphincter division) and identify areas of infection that would have been missed otherwise.

INTRODUCTION

Fistula-in-ano describes an abnormal communication between the anal (occasionally rectal) lumen and skin, usually perianal. Fistula-in-ano is relatively common and frequently recurs in the face of apparently curative surgery. Recurrence is usually due to infection that has escaped surgical detection, thereby going untreated. It is now well-recognized that preoperative MR imaging identifies fistulas and associated abscesses and extensions that would have been missed otherwise. Because of this, preoperative MR imaging has been shown to influence subsequent surgery and thereby diminish the chance of recurrence significantly. Preoperative MR imaging is routine in many centers, especially for patients with recurrent fistulas.

ETIOLOGY, CLASSIFICATION, AND TREATMENT OF FISTULA-IN-ANO

Cryptogenic fistula-in-ano is caused by chronic intersphincteric sepsis. Infection of the anal glands, which arise at the level of the dentate line (the squamocolumnar junction of the anal canal) is believed to be the initiating factor. An intersphincteric abscess results, that is, an abscess in the gap between the internal and external sphincter.[1,2] Acute glandular infection often presents as an acute perianal abscess, which is easy to diagnose clinically, and familiar to any surgical resident. Although speedy incision and drainage provides substantial symptom relief, because the abscess is underpinned by glandular infection and the gland drains to the anal lumen, patients frequently develop a subsequent fistula. Of 165,536 patients presenting with acute abscess, 16% developed a fistula subsequently, increasing to 42% if there was inflammatory bowel disease[3]; fistulas usually developed within the first year. Acute MR imaging (before incision and drainage) may show intersphincteric infection, thus identifying cryptoglandular infection as the cause (**Fig. 1**). A Cochrane review found that treatment of any underlying fistula found during surgery for acute abscess decreased the chance of recurrence substantially.[4]

Disclosure Statement: The author declares no commercial or financial conflicts of interest related to the topic discussed in this article.
UCL Department of Imaging, UCL Centre for Medical Imaging, Second Floor, Charles Bell House, 43-45 Foley Street, London W1W 7TS, UK
E-mail address: s.halligan@ucl.ac.uk

Magn Reson Imaging Clin N Am 28 (2020) 141–151
https://doi.org/10.1016/j.mric.2019.09.006

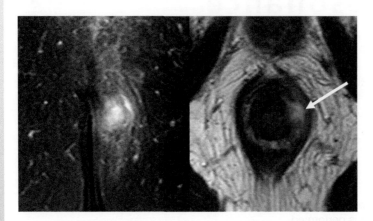

Fig. 1. Axial short T1 inversion recovery (STIR) (*left*) and T2-weighted (*right*) images in a man with acute perianal abscess. The abscess and associated inflammation are easily seen on the STIR sequence. Careful inspection shows that the inflammation (*arrow*, T2 sequence) extends into the intersphincteric plane, diagnosing anal gland infection as the underlying cause.

If intersphincteric sepsis is left untreated, it becomes chronic and burrows its way out, appearing as an external perianal opening. The anatomic course of the fistula is dictated by the location of the infected anal gland and the anatomic planes and structures that surround it. The internal opening is usually within the anal canal at the level of the dentate line, that is, the original site of the duct draining the infected gland. Radially, this is usually posterior at 6 o'clock, simply because anal glands are more abundant here, especially in men. The dentate line cannot be identified as a discrete anatomic structure by any imaging technique, but its position can be approximated with sufficient accuracy by experienced radiologists—it lies approximately 2 cm cranial to the anal verge.

The fistula can reach the skin via a variety of routes, some more tortuous than others and penetrating anal sphincter muscles and surrounding tissues to a variable degree. Fistulas are classified according to the route taken by this primary track, that is, the main track that links the internal and external openings. There are many classification systems, both clinical and radiologic, but the only system recognized commonly by surgeons is from Parks and colleagues[5] in 1976. Generally speaking, Parks' is the only system that surgeons use, which obliges radiologists to use it as well. Parks and colleagues[5] analyzed 400 consecutive fistula patients referred to St. Mark's Hospital London, a specialist hospital dealing with coloproctological disease and found that all fistulas could be placed into 1 of 4 broad groups. They termed these: intersphincteric, trans-sphincteric, suprasphincteric, and extrasphincteric (**Fig. 2**). The first 3 types pivot on intersphincteric infection, explained by the cryptoglandular hypothesis. The fourth type, extrasphincteric, does not exhibit

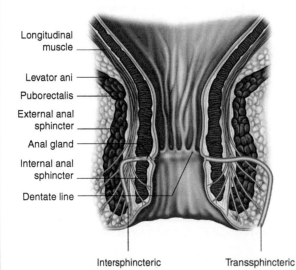
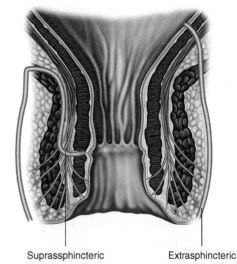

Longitudinal muscle
Levator ani
Puborectalis
External anal sphincter
Anal gland
Internal anal sphincter
Dentate line

Intersphincteric   Transsphincteric   Suprassphincteric   Extrasphincteric

Fig. 2. Coronal illustration of the anal canal showing important anatomic landmarks and the Parks classification of fistula-in-ano. (*Adapted from* Mahadevan V. The anatomy of the rectum and anal canal. Surgery 2010;29(1):8; with permission.)

intersphincteric infection and usually arises from primary disease beyond the sphincter complex, for example, rectal Crohn's disease or sigmoid diverticulitis. MR imaging has been adopted widely simply because it provides accurate preoperative classification for the surgeon. It is worth noting that, if either the external or internal opening is absent, then "sinus" is the correct description.

Although most fistulas probably start as a single primary track, unabated infection may result in ramifications (often multiple) that branch away from this, generally termed extensions. Extensions may be intersphincteric, ischioanal, or supralevator (pararectal), with either track or abscess morphology. Exactly when a track becomes an abscess and vice versa has no precise definition on imaging and the surgical community also has no generally accepted definition. The ischioanal fossa is the commonest site for an extension, especially those arising from the apex of a trans-sphincteric fistula. The ischioanal fossa lies lateral to the sphincter complex and is largely fat filled. Because this compartment lies adjacent to the anus (vs the rectum) and lies below the pelvic floor (defined by the levator plate), the author prefers the term ischioanal fossa rather than ischiorectal, which surgeons use commonly. The 2 terms are largely interchangeable. Extensions also occur in the horizontal plane, and are known as horseshoes only when there is ramification of sepsis on both sides of the internal opening. Extensions are the prime cause of recurrent disease because they are missed frequently, often left untreated, and thereby allow infection to continue. Supralevator extensions are a particular problem because the levator plate presents a relative barrier to free drainage, so that infection may persist even when the extension has been identified and incised.

So, the surgeon's prime objective is to identify the primary track and any associated extensions, eradicate these by draining all associated infection, and simultaneously preserving anal continence via minimal sphincter division. The surgeons needs answers to the following 2 questions:

- What is the relationship between the fistula and the anal sphincter? Will my surgery risk incontinence?
- Are there any extensions from the primary track that need to be treated to prevent recurrence? If so, where are they?

Surgical treatment is usually straightforward. Laying open the fistula, a procedure known as a fistulotomy, is the obvious surgical option, but risks incontinence if a substantial proportion of sphincter muscle is divided. Fistulotomy is therefore preceded by examination under (general) anesthetic (EUA), during which the surgeon attempts to classify the fistula via palpation and probing the external opening. This is not as easy as it sounds: The surgeon cannot visualize underlying muscles without incision, the internal opening may be very small and difficult to identify, the fistula may be very tortuous, and extensions may travel far from the external opening, among other considerations. Furthermore, injudicious, overenthusiastic probing can convert a simple fistula into a disaster. For example, probing the apex of a trans-sphincteric fistula could rupture through the levator plate, thereby causing a supralevator extension. Even worse, the probe can rupture into the rectum, causing an extrasphincteric fistula.

So, fistula classification by EUA alone can be very difficult, presenting ample opportunity to make matters worse. Patients with recurrent disease are particularly difficult: They are most likely to harbor extensions, but also the most difficult to assess because multiple failed previous operations results in scarring and induration that frustrates palpation. It can be extremely difficult to differentiate between an abscess or scar tissue on the basis of palpation alone. Furthermore, this group are also most likely to have extensions very remote from the primary track, frustrating their detection further. The more chronic the fistula, the more complicated the associated extensions tend to be. The inevitable result is that these patients become progressively more difficult to treat, with both patient and surgeon becoming ever more exasperated. The key to breaking this loop is accurate preoperative imaging.

If imaging suggests that extensive sphincter division will be necessary to lay open the fistula, then procedures aiming to minimize sphincter division can be deployed, but these often have a greater chance of postoperative recurrence. A variety are now available: Mucosal advancement flap is the most established and involves closing the internal opening using rectal mucosa. Newer techniques include ligation of the intersphincteric fistula tract and video-assisted anal fistula treatment, which aim to close the internal opening and eradicate intersphincteric infection while avoiding sphincter division.[6] Plugs and glue have also been inserted into the fistula to try and achieve closure without surgical incision.[6]

IMAGING FISTULA-IN-ANO: WHICH TECHNIQUE TO USE?

Before MR imaging, radiologists trying to answer the surgical questions posed elsewhere in this article met with little success. Contrast fistulography involves catheterizing the external opening with a fine cannula and injecting water-soluble contrast. It suffers 2 major drawbacks: First, extensions may fail to fill with contrast if they are plugged with debris, very remote, or if there is excessive contrast reflux from the internal and/or external openings. Second, the sphincter muscles and pelvic floor are not imaged directly, which means that the relationship between these and the fistula is largely conjecture. For example, it is frequently very difficult to decide whether a visualized extension is supralevator or in the roof of the ischioanal fossa (ie, infralevator). Ultimately, fistulography is difficult to interpret and unreliable. Initial reports of computed tomography scans were encouraging, but simple identification of the fistula is insufficient; correct classification is key. Compared with MR imaging, computed tomography scans suffer insufficient tissue contrast, especially if the fistula has not been cannulated, and its multiplanar capability also lags behind.

Anal endosonography (AES) was the first technique to visualize the anal sphincter complex with high spatial resolution and, naturally, AES has been applied to fistula classification. Although AES can be very useful, accurate interpretation depends highly on the experience of the sonographer. Also, structures remote from the endoluminal transducer are difficult to image because of limited beam penetration, especially if high frequency. Accordingly, extensions beyond the sphincter complex are missed easily and false-positive results also occur. For example, AES cannot differentiate infection or pus from fibrosis reliably, because all appear hyporeflective. This causes particular difficulties in patients with recurrent disease, because infected tracks and fibrotic scars frequently occur together. Although there is no doubt that AES is valuable in the right hands, MR imaging is superior: A study comparing AES to digital evaluation and MR imaging in 108 primary tracks found that digital evaluation in clinic correctly classified 61%, AES 81%, and MR imaging 90%.[7] Although AES was particularly adept at predicting the site of the internal opening correctly, there is little doubt that MR imaging is a superior technique overall and is certainly more generalizable.

MR Imaging Technique

MR imaging has emerged as the preeminent imaging modality to classify fistula-in-ano because it can depict infected tracks and extensions vividly and define their relationship to surrounding structures precisely. It is straightforward to image in the surgically relevant coronal plane and fistula morphology can be determined easily. The ability of MR imaging to not only accurately classify tracks but also to identify disease that would otherwise have been missed has had a palpable effect on surgical treatment and, ultimately, patient outcome[8,9]; this factor underpins its widespread adoption.

Field strength is not critical and excellent results can be obtained using relatively modest MR imaging scanners without specialized coils. Phased array surface coils increase the signal-to-noise ratio and spatial resolution to good effect,[10,11] and are generally available. Although the best spatial resolution is achieved via dedicated endoluminal anal coils,[12] these suffer the same limitation as AES—the limited field of view means that distant extensions are missed easily.[13] They are also frequently uncomfortable for the patient. So, after initial enthusiasm, they are now used rarely. It should also be stressed that endoluminal anal coils are not rectal coils; they are smaller in diameter and their active element crosses the sphincter complex, not the rectal ampulla.

The MR imaging sequences used to classify fistula-in-ano must combine anatomic precision (to determine the course of the fistula with respect to adjacent structures), with the facility to highlight sepsis (usually pus) and tissue inflammation. Many investigators use widely available fast spin echo T2-weighted sequences, which highlight the hyperintense fluid within the fistula while simultaneously discriminating the individual layers of the anal sphincter complex. Fat suppression techniques are very useful. The earliest reports used short T1 inversion recovery (STIR) imaging, with the addition of T1-weighted scans to help anatomic clarification,[14] and gadolinium contrast may be used if desired.[15] Other approaches have included saline instillation into the external opening or rectal contrast medium, but such measures increase complexity in the face of already excellent results, so there is little motivation to adopt them. For the majority of his clinical work the Author uses either 1.5 T or 3.0 T magnets and STIR/T2-weighted sequences, which makes for a very rapid and easy examination. A typical examination would comprise sagittal and axial T2-weighted acquisitions with axial and coronal STIR acquisitions.

Perhaps more important than the sequences used is the need to align the scan planes with respect to the anal sphincter axis. This is because the anal canal is tilted forwards from the vertical by approximately 45°. Straight axial and coronal images with respect to the table will provide oblique images of the sphincter complex, making the

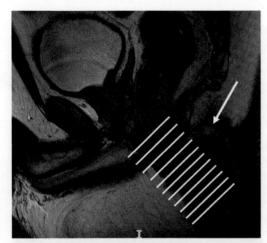

Fig. 3. Sagittal T2-weighted midline scan showing correct orientation of axial scan planes for optimal examination of the anus for fistula-in-ano. Coronal scanning is planned at 90° to these. A posterior trans-sphincteric fistula (*arrow*) is present.

geography of any fistula very difficult to ascertain. This is especially so when trying to determine the height of the internal opening. Oblique axial and coronal planes orientated orthogonal and parallel to the anal sphincter are fundamental, and planned easily from a midline sagittal image (**Fig. 3**). It may be necessary to align supplementary scans to the rectal axis for complex extrasphincteric cases with high rectal openings, but this is rare.

It is important the imaged volume extends several centimeters above the levator muscles and also includes the whole presacral space, to capture remote extensions. The entire perineum should also be included as the external opening may be beyond the immediate perianal region. Indeed, tracks may extend for several centimeters, reaching the groins or legs. Any track visible on the standard image volume should be followed to its termination. The precise location of the primary track (eg, ischioanal or intersphincteric) is usually most easily appreciated via axial images, which also best display the radial site of the internal opening. Coronal images best visualize the levator plates, that separate supralevator from infralevator disease. The height of the internal opening is also best appreciated on coronal images, with the caveat that the anal canal must be imaged along its entire craniocaudal extent, as explained.

MR Imaging Interpretation and Reporting

Active fistula tracks are filled with pus and granulation tissue, and thus appear hyperintense on T2-weighted or STIR sequences. Chronic tracks are often surrounded by a hypointense fibrous

wall, which can be relatively thick, especially in patients with recurrent disease after previous surgery. The external anal sphincter is relatively hypointense and its lateral border contrasts sharply against fat within the ischioanal fossa, especially on T2-weighted studies. Consequently, it is relatively easy to determine whether a fistula remains within the boundaries of the external sphincter or extends beyond it.

If a fistula remains contained by the external sphincter throughout its course, then it is highly likely to be intersphincteric (**Fig. 4**). In contrast, the hallmark of trans-sphincteric, suprasphincteric, and extrasphincteric fistulas is sepsis in the ischioanal fossa: It is the level of the internal opening and the level at which the primary track crosses the sphincter complex that differentiates between these types. A track in the ischioanal fossa is usually indicates a trans-sphincteric fistula (**Fig. 5**) simply because this type is much commoner than suprasphincteric or extrasphincteric classifications.

It can be difficult to identify the exact location of the internal opening. Two questions must be answered: what is its radial location and what is its craniocaudal level? The vast majority of fistulas enter the anal canal at the level of the dentate line, commensurate with the cryptoglandular hypothesis of fistula pathogenesis. Furthermore, most fistulas also enter posteriorly, at 6 o'clock, especially in men. Although the dentate line cannot be identified as a discrete anatomic entity, even

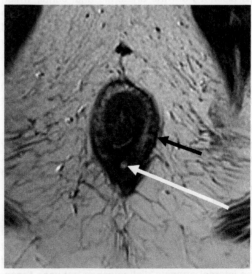

Fig. 4. Axial T2-weighted scan in a patient with an intersphincteric fistula (*white arrow*). The fistula lies within the intersphincteric plane. The lateral margin of the external sphincter (*black arrow*) is appreciated easily on MR imaging.

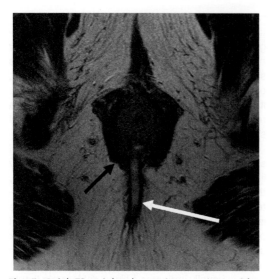

Fig. 5. Axial T2-weighted scan in a patient with a trans-sphincteric fistula (*white arrow*). The fistula track clearly lies lateral to the external sphincter boundary (*black arrow*) and penetrates the sphincter to reach a posterior internal opening at 6 o'clock, at dentate line level.

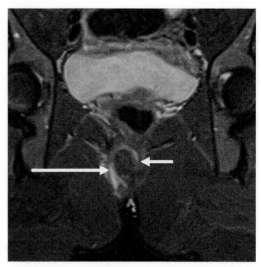

Fig. 6. Coronal STIR image of a suprasphincteric fistula (*long white arrow*). The primary track in the ischioanal fossa arches over the puborectalis to descend toward an internal opening (*short white arrow*) at dentate line level.

when using endoanal receiver coils, its general position can be estimated with sufficient precision by the experienced radiologist. The dentate line lies at approximately mid-anal canal level, which is generally midway between the superior border of the puborectalis muscle and the most caudal extent of the subcutaneous external sphincter. These landmarks define the surgical anal canal (as distinct from the anatomic anal canal, which is shorter, and defined as the canal caudal to the anal valves). The dentate level is estimated most easily using coronal views, which allow the craniocaudal extent of the puborectalis muscle and external sphincter to be appreciated. Nevertheless, its approximate location can also be estimated from axial views given sufficient experience. It should be noted that in many patients the puborectalis muscle is rather gracile, quite unlike the bulky muscle depicted in many anatomic textbooks. Notably, the puborectalis frequently blends imperceptibly into the deep external sphincter, which hampers precise identification of mid-anal canal level on imaging. Again, this can be overcome with experience. Any fistula track that penetrates the pelvic floor above the level of the puborectalis muscle is potentially suprasphincteric or extrasphincteric. The level of the internal opening distinguishes between these, being anal in the former (**Fig. 6**) and rectal in the latter (**Fig. 7**).

Trans-sphincteric fistulas penetrate the external sphincter directly, a feature that can be easily

appreciated on axial or coronal views (see **Fig. 5**). MR imaging has revealed that a trans-sphincteric track may cross the sphincter at a variety of angles.[16] For example, it may arch upward as it passes through the external sphincter, thus

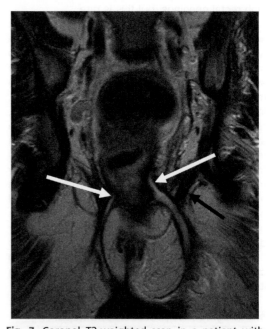

Fig. 7. Coronal T2-weighted scan in a patient with bilateral extrasphincteric fistulas (*white arrows*). The internal opening for each fistula is directly into the distal rectum, well above the level of the levator plate (*black arrow*), which indicates pelvic floor level.

crossing the muscle at a higher level than would be anticipated merely from inspecting the level of the internal opening. This is important because such tracks require a greater degree of sphincter incision if fistulotomy is performed, with a correspondingly increased risk of postoperative incontinence. Coronal MR imaging is best able to estimate the precise angulation of the track with respect to the surrounding sphincter.[16]

The radial site of the internal opening is simple to identify if the fistula track can be traced right to the anal mucosa but this is unusual because the internal opening is rarely widely patent; rather, it is usually compressed and can be very difficult to see directly. In most cases, intelligent deduction is all that is needed; the internal opening is likely to lie in the region of maximal intersphincteric sepsis. The intersphincteric space lies between the internal and external sphincter and contains the longitudinal muscle, which often seems to be rather fragmented. The internal sphincter is hyperintense on both T2-weighted fast spin echo and STIR sequences.

Extensions

The major advantage of MR imaging is the ease with which it identifies extensions associated with the primary track. Like tracks, extensions manifest as hyperintense regions on T2-weighted and STIR imaging, and their margins also enhance further following intravenous contrast. Like the primary track, collateral inflammation can be present

to variable extent. The commonest type of extension is one arising from the apex of a transsphincteric track, extending into the roof of the ipsilateral ischioanal fossa (**Fig. 8**). The major benefit of preoperative MR imaging is that it alerts the surgeon to extensions that would otherwise be missed at EUA. This is especially the case when extensions are either contralateral to the primary track or are several centimeters remote from it. It is especially important to image supralevator extensions (**Fig. 9**) because these are both difficult for the surgeon to detect and pose specific difficulties with treatment because of their location above the pelvic floor.

Horseshoe extensions are recognized by their unique semilunar configuration (**Fig. 10**). Strictly speaking, sepsis should extend on both sides of the internal opening for a correct diagnosis of a horseshoe. Horseshoes may be intersphincteric, ischioanal, or supralevator. As emphasized previously, complex extensions are especially common in patients with recurrent fistula-in-ano and/or those who have Crohn's disease.

The Radiologic Report

The author reports his MR imaging studies as follows: The clinical details that accompany the referral are stated first. This is followed by the fistula classification and its radial or quadrantic location. The radial site of the enteric communication is stated along with its level. The location of the

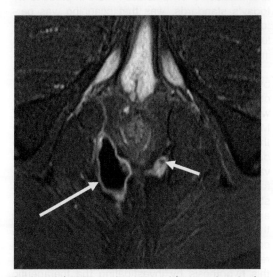

Fig. 8. Axial STIR scan in a man with extensions in the roof of both ischioanal fossae. The left-sided extension contains a seton thread (*short white arrow*). The right-sided extension (*long white arrow*) is predominantly gas filled, indicating that it is well-drained.

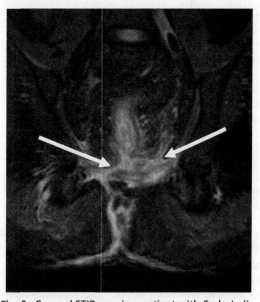

Fig. 9. Coronal STIR scan in a patient with Crohn's disease and an extrasphincteric fistula. There is extensive bilateral sepsis (*white arrows*) above the level of the pelvic floor.

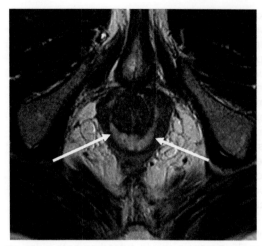

Fig. 10. Axial T2-weighted scan in a patient with a horseshoe extension (*white arrows*). The extension lies medial to the external sphincter and puborectalis, confirming sepsis in the intersphincteric and supralevator compartments.

external opening is mentioned (although this is usually obvious to the surgeon on clinical inspection). A statement is then made regarding extensions, that is, whether there are any associated present or not and, if so, the anatomic compartment (intersphincteric, ischioanal, supralevator), and radial location. This procedure is repeated for each individual fistula if multiple and a statement made regarding the relationship between multiple fistulas, for example, do some share a common internal opening, which structures do they communicate across? A statement is then made regarding comparison to previous imaging, if this is available. It is not useful to describe the many twists and turns of each individual fistula because this is not how colorectal surgeons conceptualize fistula-in-ano; use the Parks classification so that the report is in a language that they understand. An example of a recent report by the author is as follows: "Clinical details: Anal fistula ?classification. Findings: There is a transsphincteric fistula in the right posterior quadrant at 5 o'clock with an internal opening at 6 o'clock at dentate line level. There are 2 extensions: The first is in the roof of the ipsilateral ischioanal fossa, just subjacent to the levator plate; the second is a cranial intersphincteric extension at 3 o'clock that terminates in a 2 cm left-sided supralevator abscess. Conclusion: Complex trans-sphincteric fistula with ipsilateral supra- and infralevator extensions as described above." That is a fairly brief report in terms of words, but one that describes a very complex fistula in language that a competent colorectal surgeon will understand and,

importantly, alerts him or her to the surgical issues that they will face at subsequent EUA.

EFFECT OF PREOPERATIVE MR IMAGING ON SURGERY AND SUBSEQUENT CLINICAL OUTCOME

Over the last 20 years, MR imaging has revolutionized the treatment of patients with fistula-in-ano. As stated, this is because MR imaging can classify fistulas preoperatively with very high accuracy and, in doing so, alerts the surgeon to disease that might otherwise have been missed. Although there are MR imaging reports in radiologic journals dating from 1989,[17] it was not until the seminal description by Lunniss and coworkers[14] that the true potential of MR imaging was appreciated fully by a surgical audience. Lunniss and associates imaged 16 patients with cryptoglandular fistula-in-ano and compared the MR imaging classification with that from subsequent EUA. MR imaging agreed with EUA in 14 of the 16 cases (88%), confirming immediately that it was by far the most accurate preoperative assessment available. In the remaining 2 patients, MR imaging had suggested disease but EUA was normal. Two months later, both patients re-presented with disease at the site initially indicated by MR imaging. The clear implication was that EUA had missed disease, not MR imaging. This led the authors to conclude that, "MR imaging is the most accurate method for determining the presence and course of anal fistulae."[14] What is even more impressive by today's standards, was that scanning was performed at 0.5 T, suggesting clearly that high resolution and other factors are unnecessary for MR imaging to be clinically useful.

Lunnis' excellent results were confirmed rapidly by others, and then elaborated on. Spencer and colleagues[18] classified 37 patients into those with simple or complex fistulas on the basis of MR imaging and EUA independently. They found that imaging was the better predictor of clinical outcome, with positive and negative predictive values of 73% versus 57% and 87% versus 64% for MR imaging and surgery, respectively. This study provided compelling evidence that MR imaging was related more closely to clinical outcome than EUA, indicating that preoperative MR imaging could identify features that caused postoperative recurrence. Beets-Tan and colleagues[10] extended this hypothesis by investigating the therapeutic impact of MR imaging; preoperative findings in 56 patients were revealed to the operating surgeon after they had completed an initial EUA. MR imaging provided important additional information that precipitated further surgery in 12 of 56 patients

(21%), mostly in those with recurrent fistulas or Crohn's disease.[10] Buchanan and coworkers[11] therefore hypothesized that the therapeutic impact and consequent beneficial effect of preoperative MR imaging would be greatest in patients with recurrent fistulas, since these were most likely to harbor occult infection while simultaneously being the most difficult to evaluate clinically. After an initial EUA, they revealed the findings of preoperative MR imaging in 71 patients with recurrent fistulas. The surgeon was then free to act on the MR imaging findings as they saw fit, EUA completed, and the clinical course of each individual patient followed subsequently. They found that postoperative recurrence was 16% for those surgeons who always acted when MR imaging suggested they had missed areas of sepsis. In contrast, recurrence was 57% for those surgeons who always chose to ignore imaging, believing their own assessment to be superior.[11] Furthermore, of the 16 patients who needed further unplanned surgery, MR imaging correctly predicted the site of recurrent disease in all cases.[11]

Ever since Lunnis' work suggested that EUA might not be as accurate as MR imaging,[14] comparative studies have been plagued by the lack of a genuine reference standard. It is now well-recognized that surgical findings at EUA are often incorrect. In particular, false-negative diagnoses at EUA are relatively frequent. In a recent comparative study of endosonography, MR imaging and EUA in 34 patients with fistulas owing to Crohn's disease, Schwartz and co-workers[19] found that a combination of results from at least 2 modalities was necessary for the classification to be correct. Because surgical false negatives only reveal themselves over the course of long-term clinical follow-up, comparative studies that ignore clinical outcome are likely to be seriously flawed. Recognizing this, Buchanan and co-workers[7] examined 108 primary fistula tracks by digital examination, AES, and MR imaging, and then followed patients' clinical progress to establish an enhanced reference standard for each patient that was based on ultimate clinical outcome rather than EUA. The authors found that digital evaluation correctly classified 61% of primary tracks, AES 81%, and MR imaging 90%.[7] Although endosonography was particularly adept at predicting the site of the internal opening correctly, achieving this in 91%, MR imaging was even better at 97%. Indeed, MR imaging was superior to endosonography in all assessments investigated by the authors.[7] Although endosonography is undoubtedly a useful tool to classify fistula-in-ano, it cannot compete with MR imaging, especially for detection of extensions, which is

undoubtedly the most important role for preoperative imaging. Furthermore, MR imaging is also more generally available and less operator dependent.

DIFFERENTIAL DIAGNOSIS OF PERIANAL SEPSIS

Not all perianal sepsis is caused by fistula-in-ano. For example, acne conglobata, hidradenitis suppurativa, pilonidal sinus, actinomycosis, tuberculosis, proctitis, human immunodeficiency virus infection, lymphoma, and anal and rectal carcinoma may all cause perianal infection. Although clinical examination is often conclusive, this is not always so and imaging helps frequently with the differential diagnosis. As discussed elsewhere in this article, the cardinal feature of fistula-in-ano is intersphincteric infection, which is not generally found in other conditions, although it may be detected if MR imaging is used to image acute anorectal abscesses. Whenever imaging suggests that infection is superficial rather than deep seated, and that there is no sphincteric involvement, then other conditions such as hidradenitis suppurativa should be considered.[20] For example, a study comparing patients with pilonidal sinus (Fig. 11) and fistula-in-ano found that MR imaging could reliably distinguish between the two on the basis of intersphincteric infection and an enteric

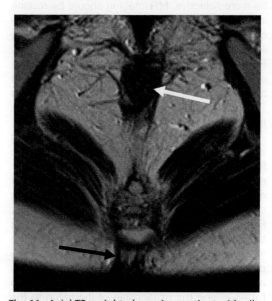

Fig. 11. Axial T2-weighted scan in a patient with pilonidal sinus. The sinus (*black arrow*) manifests as an infected pit in the subcutaneous tissues overlying the coccyx. There is no communication with the anal sphincter complex. In particular, there is no sepsis in the intersphincteric plane (*white arrow*).

opening, both of which were always absent in pilonidal sinus.[21]

The possibility of underlying Crohn's disease should always be considered in patients who have particularly complex fistulas, especially if the history is relatively short. Indeed, a perianal fistula is the presenting symptom in approximately 5% of Crohn's patients and up to 40% experience anal disease over the course of their disease.[22] MR imaging examination can be extended cranially to encompass the small bowel if Crohn's disease is suspected and the possibility of underlying pelvic disease should be considered in any patient with an extrasphincteric fistula, whether thought to be due to Crohn's disease or not.

WHICH PATIENTS SHOULD BE IMAGED?

Although most patients with fistula-in-ano are simple to both diagnose and treat, a significant proportion will benefit from preoperative MR imaging. Where MR imaging is accessed easily, it could be argued that all patients should be imaged preoperatively. Supporting this, although the therapeutic impact of MR imaging is greatest in patients with complex disease,[9,10] it has been estimated that MR imaging benefits around 10% of patients presenting for the first time with seemingly simple fistulas, but who ultimately prove to be more complex.[23] Where MR imaging access is more restricted, the referring clinician needs to be more selective. MR imaging should be routine in patients with recurrent disease, because evidence that MR imaging alters surgical therapy and improves clinical outcome is overwhelming. Patients presenting for the first time with a fistula appearing complex on clinical examination should also be referred, as should patients with known Crohn's disease since the prevalence of complex fistulas is so high.

There are also surgical situations where imaging is likely to be particularly beneficial, even when the fistula itself is simple. For example, the anterior external sphincter is very short in women and dividing this during fistulotomy risks postoperative incontinence, even when the fistula is simple. Faced with such a dilemma, rather than incising the fistula the surgeon may choose to pass a seton thread through the track to stimulate drainage. The patient can then be imaged postoperatively to assess the potential extent of sphincter division by visualizing the relationship of the seton to the external sphincter. A decision can then be made whether to progress with fistulotomy or to keep the seton in place for a few months, after which time the internal opening can be closed with a rectal mucosal advancement flap or another sphincter-saving procedure. Setons may also be placed at EUA when the surgeon is uncertain about the relationship between the track and the sphincter, and then imaged postoperatively to answer this question (especially if MR imaging was not performed beforehand).

The benefit of MR imaging is not restricted to surgical assessment. The advent of monoclonal antibody to human tumor necrosis factor alpha has impacted dramatically upon the medical management of patients with Crohn's fistulas. However, therapy is contraindicated if an abscess is present (because this can be associated with overwhelming sepsis) and MR imaging is useful to search for this. Indeed, MR imaging is now frequently used to monitor therapy because it has shown that fistulas may persist in the face of clinical findings suggesting remission. An early MR imaging study of patients whose external opening has closed revealed that deeper sepsis often persisted, indicating that therapy should continue.[24]

CONCLUSION

In patients with fistula-in-ano who have a high likelihood of complex disease, the evidence that preoperative MR imaging influences the surgical approach, extent of exploration, and improves ultimate outcome is overwhelming. The author hopes that this article stimulates more surgeons to ask this service from their radiologists, and for radiologists to provide it. Doing so will reduce the incidence of recurrent fistula-in-ano and the misery it causes.

Future Directions

Multiple peer-reviewed, indexed studies have proven that MR imaging classification of fistula-in-ano is highly accurate in the right hands. Given that MR imaging is already so effective, the incentive to further develop the technique is relatively limited and research in this specific area has slowed over the last decade. Nevertheless, workers are investigating whether the degree and nature of dynamic enhancement is able to provide prognostic information regarding disease trajectory in patients with Crohn's disease[25] and large randomized trials of the various new surgical therapies now available (eg, the FIAT trial, ISRCTN78352529) will provide the substrate for further research given that MR imaging is now embedded in these as the reference standard for fistula healing.

SUMMARY

Preoperative MR imaging is undoubtedly the most effective method with which to classify fistula-in-ano and is especially useful for complex cases, where its ability to identify remote and unsuspected extensions has considerable therapeutic impact. Postoperative recurrence is reduced when surgeons act on MR imaging findings, thereby avoiding the misery that this disease causes for patients.

ACKNOWLEDGMENTS

The author is funded by the UK National Institute for Health Research via the University College London Hospitals Biomedical Research Centre.

REFERENCES

1. Chiari H. Uber die analen divertikel der rectumschleimhaut und ihre beziehung zu den anal fisteln, vol. 19. Austria: Wien Med Press; 1878. p. 1482–3.
2. Parks AG. The pathogenesis and treatment of fistula-in-ano. Br Med J 1961;5224:463–9.
3. Sahnan K, Askari A, Adegbola SO, et al. Natural history of anorectal sepsis. Br J Surg 2017;104: 1857–65.
4. Malik AI, Nelson RL, Tou S. Incision and drainage of perianal abscess with or without treatment of anal fistula. Cochrane Database Syst Rev 2010;(7): CD006827.
5. Parks AG, Gordon PH, Hardcastle JD. A classification of fistula –in-ano. Br J Surg 1976;63:1–12.
6. Limura E, Giordano P. Modern management of anal fistula. World J Gastroenterol 2015;21:12–20.
7. Buchanan G, Halligan S, Bartram CI, et al. Clinical examination, endosonography, and magnetic resonance imaging for preoperative assessment of fistula-in-ano: comparison to an outcome derived reference standard. Radiology 2004;233:674–81.
8. Halligan S, Buchanan G. Imaging fistula-in-ano. Eur J Radiol 2003;42:98–107.
9. Halligan S, Stoker J. Imaging fistula-in-ano: state-of-the-art. Radiology 2006;239:18–33.
10. Beets-Tan RG, Beets GL, van der Hoop AG, et al. Preoperative MR imaging of anal fistulas: does it really help the surgeon? Radiology 2001;218: 75–84.
11. Buchanan G, Halligan S, Williams A, et al. Effect of MRI on clinical outcome of recurrent fistula-in-ano. Lancet 2002;360:1661–2.
12. Hussain SM, Stoker J, Schouten WR, et al. Fistula in ano: endoanal sonography versus endoanal MR imaging in classification. Radiology 1996;200: 475–81.
13. Halligan S, Bartram CI. MR imaging of fistula in ano: are endoanal coils the gold standard? AJR Am J Roentgenol 1998;171:407–12.
14. Lunniss PJ, Armstrong P, Barker PG, et al. Magnetic resonance imaging of anal fistulae. Lancet 1992; 340:394–6.
15. Spencer JA, Ward J, Beckingham IJ, et al. Dynamic contrast-enhanced MR imaging of perianal fistulas. Am J Roentgenol 1996;167:735–41.
16. Buchanan GN, Williams AB, Bartram CI, et al. Potential clinical implications of direction of a transsphincteric anal fistula track. Br J Surg 2003;90: 1250–5.
17. Koelbel G, Schmiedl U, Majer MC, et al. Diagnosis of fistulae and sinus tracts in patients with Crohn disease: value of MR imaging. Am J Roentgenol 1989;152:999–1003.
18. Spencer JA, Chapple K, Wilson D, et al. Outcome after surgery for perianal fistula: predictive value of MR imaging. Am J Roentgenol 1998; 171:403–6.
19. Schwartz DA, Wiersema MJ, Dudiak KM, et al. A comparison of endoscopic ultrasound, magnetic resonance imaging, and exam under anesthesia for evaluation of Crohn's perianal fistulas. Gastroenterology 2001;121:1064–72.
20. Griffin N, Williams AB, Anderson S, et al. Hidradenitis suppurativa: MRI features in anogenital disease. Dis Colon Rectum 2014;57:762–71.
21. Taylor SA, Halligan S, Bartram CI. Pilonidal sinus disease: MR imaging distinction from fistula in ano. Radiology 2003;226:662–7.
22. Schwartz DA, Loftus EV Jr, Tremaine WJ, et al. The natural history of fistulizing Crohn's disease in Olmsted County, Minnesota. Gastroenterology 2002;122:875–80.
23. Buchanan GN, Halligan S, Williams AB, et al. Magnetic resonance imaging for primary fistula in ano. Br J Surg 2003;90:877–81.
24. Bell SJ, Halligan S, Windsor ACJ, et al. Response of fistulating Crohn's disease to infliximab treatment assessed by magnetic resonance imaging. Aliment Pharmacol Ther 2003; 17:387–93.
25. Horsthuis K, Lavini C, Bipat S, et al. Perianal Crohn disease: evaluation of dynamic contrast enhanced MR imaging as an indicator of disease activity. Radiology 2009;251:380–7.